GMAT®

PRACTICE EXAMINATIONS

E M ROMER BS MS EAA MA
J C GARVER BA MA PhD
W M STEVENSON MA PhD

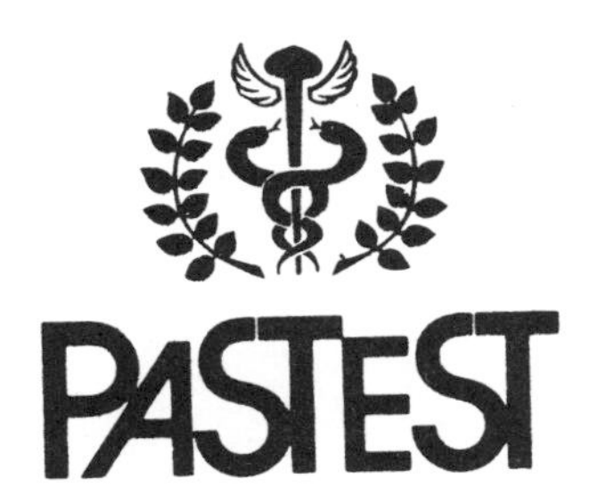

PASTEST

PASTEST
Rankin House, Parkgate Estate
Knutsford
Cheshire, WA16 8DX
England

First published 1988
Reprinted 1989
Revised 1991
Reprinted 1991
Reprinted 1992
Reprinted 1994

British Library Cataloguing in Publication Data

Romer, Eugene M.
GMAT Practice Examinations.

1. Business education — Examinations, questions, etc.
I. Garver, Joseph C.; Stevenson, Winifred M. — joint authors.
II. Title
658'.007'11

ISBN 0-906896-36-3

Acknowledgement

GMAT is a registered trademark of the Graduate Management Admission Council (GMAC). The GMAT name is used with permission by GMAC, but its use does not constitute an endorsement by GMAC. The GMAC has also given permission to use instructions and format similar to the GMAT but has neither provided nor approved the material herein.

Printed and bound in Great Britain by Biddles Limited, Guildford and King's Lynn

CONTENTS

INTRODUCTION

In this book, you will find two practice examinations for the Graduate Management Admission Test (GMAT). At the end of each examination, correct answers and explanations have been provided. At the back of the book, there is a computer answer sheet for you to record your answers.

The official GMAT examination consists of seven sections, each of 30 minutes duration. Of these, only six sections contribute to your scores. Included in the seven sections is one section containing trial or experimental questions used for pre-testing and equating purposes. Although these trial questions are not scored, the trial section is not identified and candidates taking the actual GMAT examination normally will not be able to distinguish the trial section from the questions that will be scored. It is important that you approach all questions as if they will contribute to the final score.

In this book, there are two complete examinations, each containing six sections, but all sections in each examination are designed to contribute to your scores.

Particular efforts have been made to follow the style, content, and format of the official examination in order to provide as much appropriate practice as possible. However, because the style and content of the official examination is subject to change without notice, the authors can not be held responsible for any differences between the style and format of the practice examinations and that of the official examination that may have occurred after the publication of this book. Portions of this book contain materials that are more difficult than some recent GMAT examinations. This has been done intentionally to provide the student with practice on more difficult variants of the GMAT that may be encountered. American English has been used throughout, and reading passages have been taken from U. S. sources.

THE MARKING SERVICE

A marking service is available to those who wish to take these tests under timed conditions. After we receive your computer sheets, your answers will be scored, using the same method as used on the actual examinations. You will then be sent your overall score, sub-scores, and percentile rankings for the mathematical and verbal sections of the examinations. [NOTE: If you intend to send your results to us for marking, do not use any explanatory material to change your answers. If you do so, the scoring process will be invalidated.] To make use of the marking service, simply send your completed answer forms, together with a self-addressed envelope which will be used to return your score to you, to:

PasTest
Rankin House
Parkgate Estate
KNUTSFORD
Cheshire
WA16 8DX
England

TEST-TAKING SUGGESTIONS

General suggestions -

Before you begin the examination, ensure that you know and understand the instructions that are provided at the beginning of each of the five types of question in this examination, i. e., Reading Comprehension, Sentence Correction, Critical Reasoning, Problem Solving and Data Sufficiency. (The complete set of instructions for each type can be found in the GMAT Bulletin of Information.) This knowledge will prevent you wasting time during the examination. You should also be aware that all questions are in multiple-choice format and that you are expected to choose the best answer to a question. Within any one section, the questions are designed to test either verbal skills or basic mathematical skills. All questions have equal value.

In each section, survey the questions initially and then answer the easiest questions first. The questions are designed so that most of them can be answered within a minute or two; working too long on any one question is poor test technique.

Both speed and accuracy are needed for high scores but accuracy is the more important of the two. You do not need to answer all questions to obtain a high score, e. g., if 25% of all questions were omitted in order to ensure that all the remaining questions were answered correctly, the score obtained would rank the candidate among the top 5-6% of all those taking the examination.

Guessing at random is unlikely to improve your score; the scoring method used is designed to eliminate any advantage gained through random guessing. However, if you can eliminate at least one of the choices offered, your likelihood of guessing the correct answer is improved and it may be to your advantage to take a guess at one of the remaining choices.

Specific suggestions -

The verbal sections test comprehension, your understanding of standard American written usage, and critical reasoning. Where textual materials are given, careful reading of both texts and questions is necessary to find the correct answer. Vocabulary is of primary importance; e. g., when the words imply and infer appear in the questions, they are not synonyms and may not be interchanged. In some cases, a question may be framed in such a way that the correct answer will reverse the statement as given in the text; this applies particularly to questions in which four of the options can be traced back to the text, but the required answer is the exception.

A Reading Comprehension section, with a total of twenty-five questions, will include three passages: one from each of three areas, i. e., the social sciences, the humanities, and the biological or physical sciences. Each passage is about 500 words long, followed by seven to nine questions on the material in the passage. The texts are taken from American academic sources, such as books and periodicals. All are of equal difficulty even though you may feel that one particular passage is "easier" than another. Work on the "easiest" passage first; leave the most "difficult" passage for last.

Careful examination of the texts is essential; the answer is always to be found in the passage. The questions fall into six categories, involving, (1), the overall theme of the passage — what is the passage about? (2), supporting ideas that substantiate or develop the main theme — these may be implicit rather than explicit, (3), the logical structure of the passage, describing how it is organized,

(4), the style and tone of the passage, using deduction often based on the author's choice of words, (5), analogues with the information given applied to comparable situations outside the text, and (6), inferences that can be drawn from the text, either from the theme as a whole or from some part of it.

Of the five choices offered, only one exactly matches question to answer. Sometimes the answer "translates" the text, and the translation will almost certainly have reference to the basic meanings of the words in the text, so that etymologies are significant. Where style is in question, the answer may involve some form of value judgement. A good general vocabulary is essential, and the exam requires meticulous attention to correct usage.

The Sentence Correction section tests your awareness of standard American written grammatical and idiomatic usage. Each question consists of one sentence with all or part of it underlined; only the the underlined portion may be considered for possible change. Of the five choices offered as answers, the first choice always exactly repeats the underlined portion of the question: if the sentence is correct as it stands, then the first answer will be the correct choice. If there is a mistake, it may be in the wrong use of a word or words, but much more commonly the error will be in the syntax. There are many possibilities here - wrong verb forms, wrong sequences, mismatching of pronouns, failure to observe idiomatic usage of prepositions, or confusion of different constructions. The best version is the simplest version that satisfies standard grammatical usage - the preferred version does not have changes if these are not strictly necessary. While a choice with a short answer will be preferred to a longer construction, the shortest choice is not always the correct answer because objectionable features may have been introduced.

The Critical Reasoning section, consisting of twenty questions, tests your ability to identify appropriate conclusions, underlying assumptions, parallels between analogous arguments, factors that weaken or strengthen a given argument, effectiveness of particular plans of action, and reasoning errors. In this section, each question may consist of one or two statements upon which you will have to base your choice. In some cases, there may be two questions based on a given set of statements. Each question will be based on the theme of the statement(s) made and the information presented may come in different forms — actual data, conjecture, hypothesis, even unsupported hearsay. If there is some form of argument, the conflicting views will have to be identified. "Hard facts" are always likely to be relevant to the correct answer, although the answer may require judgement or evaluation. The clues are always in the text.

The mathematical sections fall into one of two categories: problem-solving or data sufficiency. In all questions, diagrams are drawn as accurately as possible unless stated otherwise. In problems with the comment: "Note: Figure not drawn to scale," the figure is always distorted in some way; often, redrawing the figure to fit the problem statement will help simplify the analysis. Generally, the use of auxiliary diagrams to illustrate possible interactions between parts of a problem is helpful.

Do not spend too much time on any one question; most problems can be answered i a minute or two. If you are tempted to use time-consuming procedures or complicated analyses, it may be wiser to skip the question in favor of other problems that will not absorb so much time.

The two Problem-Solving sections, containing twenty questions each, are designed to test your understanding of elementary concepts of arithmetic, algebra, and geometry. Long or formal mathematical analyses are generally unnecessary; often, a simplified or approximated approach will be all that is necessary to identify the best answer.

In the Data Sufficiency section, which consists of twenty-five questions, you are tested on your ability to determine either what information is relevant to the problem or at what point sufficient information has been presented to solve the problem. For each question, you are given some information and a question to be answered. Up to this point, however, there is never sufficient information to answer the question. Following this, two auxiliary data statements are presented and your analysis is to be based on whether the first of these statements by itself, the second statement by itself, or both statements together will suffice to answer the question. For these types of questions, it may be unnecessary to work through a a problem entirely; attempts to carry out unnecessary analyses merely waste time.

A common source of error is the unintentional conflation of the first auxiliary statement with the second auxiliary statement when the second statement is supposed to be examined on its own. Additionally, errors often arise when a student assumes the existence of data that have not been explicitly stated in the question.

Further details about the examination can be found in the GMAT Bulletin of Information, which must be read very carefully.

INSTRUCTIONS

This book is divided into two complete practice examinations, and each contains six sections.

If these examinations are to give you practice under simulated examination conditions and if your score is to be a fair measure of your ability, you must follow the directions given below:

(1) Each examination requires a total of 3 hours and 10 minutes, and you should do the entire examination at one time. Therefore, you should plan to take each examination at a time when you will be undisturbed for 3 hours and 10 minutes. You may take a 10 minute break midway through the examination (at the end of the third section). Using more than the allocated time invalidates the scoring process.

(2) Each examination contains 6 sections, and these must be done in the order presented. Do not spend more than 30 minutes on any one section. If you have time to spare before the 30 minutes has expired, you may not use this spare time to work on any other section.

(3) Do not obtain help from books, notes or other people during the examination. You may not use calculators, slide rules, tables of formulae, or any other computing device in the examination.

(4) Mark your answers on the answer sheet using a Grade HB (No. 2) pencil. Have several sharpened pencils available before you start.

Use the answer sheet while you are taking the examination. You should use only the book for your working notes, as you will not be permitted to bring blank paper into the examination room to use in the actual examination. Mark your answers on the computer sheet, making certain that your mark fills the oval completely; if you wish to change an answer, make sure that you erase the wrong mark completely. If there are more spaces for answers than there are questions, the extra spaces should be ignored.

The FIRST EXAMINATION begins on the next page.

The SECOND EXAMINATION begins on page 52.

Please read the instructions carefully before working on either examination.

YOU MAY BEGIN WHEN YOU ARE READY.

Section I

Time - 30 minutes

25 Questions

<u>Directions:</u> Each passage in this group is followed by questions on content. After reading a passage, choose the best answer to each question and blacken the corresponding space on the answer sheet. Answer all questions following a passage on the basis of what is <u>stated</u> or <u>implied</u> in that passage.

Members of the folic acid group of vitamins, which are necessary for the formation of blood cells in man, include folacin (or pteroylglutamic acid), pteroyltriglutamic acid, pteroylheptaglutamic acid, and folinic acid or citrovorum factor, a derivative of folic acid that occurs in natural (5) materials in both free and combined form. Information is meager concerning the amounts of folacin and folinic acid compounds in foods and their biological availability. Enzymes that can break down conjugated pteroylglutamates (combined forms of folic acid) to folacin occur in many animal tissues. In several natural products, these enzymes or conjugases (10) are accompanied by an inhibitor. This inhibitor appears to influence the availability of the combined forms of folacin to human subjects. These findings illustrate the difficulties involved in estimating the folacin that is available from foods and in determining the human need for it.

The best sources of folacin include liver, dry beans, lentils, (15) cowpeas, asparagus, broccoli, spinach, and collards. However, intestinal bacteria synthesize folacin. This source may be important in man, because experimental deficiency has not been induced by diets low in folacin. The dietary requirement of folacin is not known, but available evidence suggests that approximately 0.1 to 0.2 milligram daily may suffice.

(20) Much has been learned about the function of folacin and its derivatives, although their exact metabolic role has not been delineated. It seems likely that a derivative of folinic acid is the functioning form of the vitamin, and that this derivative combines with a protein and functions as a coenzyme. Folacin participates in the formation by the body of complex (25) chemical compounds known as purines and pyrimidines that are utilized in the building up of nucleoproteins — that is, proteins that are found in the nucleus of every cell. The essentiality of folacin for hematopoiesis (the manufacture of blood cells) in man presumably resides in its function in the formation of purines and pyrimidines. Folic acid stimulates the formation (30) of normal blood cells in certain anemias, which are characterized by oversized red cells and the accumulation in the bone marrow of immature red blood cells called megaloblasts. The bone marrow cannot complete the manufacture of blood cells in the absence of folic acid. Cyanocobalamin is also needed for the formation of blood cells, as well as for the manufacture (35) of nucleoproteins, but the exact biochemical interrelationships of these two vitamins have not been clarified.

Two human anemias appear to be due primarily to folacin deficiency — macrocytic anemia of pregnancy and megaloblastic anemia of infancy. These anemias occasionally respond to treatment with cyanocobalamin. Macrocytic (40) anemia of pregnancy may be related to an increased folacin requirement that is not met by the diet. The syndrome of folacin deficiency in man is exemplified best by the symptoms that develop when large amounts of a folic acid antagonist such as aminopterin are administered. Manifestations include glossitis (a sore, red, smooth tongue), diarrhea, gastro-intestinal (45) lesions, and anemia. Similar symptoms occur in sprue and nutritional macrocytic anemia; these symptoms often disappear following folacin therapy.

GO ON TO THE NEXT PAGE

1. In this passage the author's main purpose is to

(A) discuss the role of the folic acid group in the therapy of human deficiency diseases
(B) outline the processes by which folacin may promote metabolism in the human body
(C) delineate the structure and function of folacin
(D) explain why the folic acid group is essential for the human body
(E) analyze the biochemical properties of folacin

2. This passage was most probably extracted from

(A) a textbook of nutritional science
(B) a textbook of biochemistry
(C) a pamphlet issued for the use of farmers
(D) an article in a journal of molecular biology
(E) a report to a congress of pathologists

3. It may be inferred from the passage that aminopterin (line 43)

(A) is a direct cause of glossitis and gastro-intestinal lesions
(B) is a synthetic enzyme (coenzyme) or conjugase
(C) causes dietary deficiency in man
(D) is a drug which counteracts folacin
(E) contributes to the development of sprue and nutritional macrocytic anemia

4. Which of the following statements is supported by the passage?

(A) folacin may play a role in the development of some forms of anemia
(B) certain human organs can synthesize folacin
(C) the human body may be unable to assimilate the folacin found in food
(D) folacin is a constituent of red blood cells
(E) folacin is a derivative of folinic acid

5. The passage contains information that answers which of the following questions?

I. Where is hematopoiesis localized?

II. What role does cyanocobalamin play in the formation of purines?

III. What is the result of a lack of folacin in the human body?

(A) I only
(B) I and II only
(C) III only
(D) I and III only
(E) I, II, and III

6. The author's presentation of his evidence and conclusions could best be described as

(A) subtle
(B) equivocal
(C) biased
(D) unquestioning
(E) cautious

GO ON TO THE NEXT PAGE

7. It can be inferred from the passage that the "diets low in folacin" mentioned in line 17

(A) resulted from an extensive agricultural failure
(B) were part of a research project in human nutrition
(C) were also deficient in cyanocobalamin
(D) must also have included large amounts of an inhibitor
(E) must have resulted in the development of anemia

8. According to the passage, the consumption of foods containing large amounts of folacin does not ensure protection against anemia, because

(A) only intestinal bacteria can synthesize folacin
(B) enzymes in animal tissue naturally break down folic acids
(C) a substance present in food seems to interfere with the assimilation of folacin
(D) the metabolic role of folacin does not preclude deficiency in the red blood cells
(E) these foods may not contain cyanocobalamin

The immediate reason for Roger Williams' expulsion from the Massachusetts Bay Colony in 1636 was that he had persisted in defying the authority of a state whose hierarchical structure depended upon obedience and unquestioning respect. Williams had presumed to contradict the decrees of the authorities (5) both temporal and spiritual, had continued to preach from his pulpit after having been solemnly forbidden to do so, and thus had been infecting others with his defiance. Dexter, the historian of Congregationalism, notes that Williams' "banishment" resulted from his "seditious, defiant, and pernicious posture toward the state." By continuing to broadcast his heterodox notions (10) on religion and government, Williams was compounding heresy and insolence, for in Massachusetts, as in Renaissance Europe, heresy was largely contempt of holy councils.

Yet, even if Williams had comported himself more discreetly, his leading ideas would inevitably have gotten him expelled, for these ideas were both (15) embarrassing and heretical, calling into question the foundation and ordering of Puritan society in the colony. Thus, on grounds of strict truthfulness, he denounced the colony's royal charter, because it contained James I's claim to have discovered the New World. Williams' absolute refusal to compromise on matters of principle led to his rejection of <u>any</u> (20) sanctified communion with either "unregenerate" persons or members of "false" churches; therefore, he opposed compulsory church attendance and even the administration of oaths to those not confirmed as God's children. Seeking to purify Puritanism, he came to advocate a total separation of church and state, including abolition of the requirement that magistrates — the (25) political officers of the colony — be "visible saints," i.e., members of the Congregationalist Church, the only church permitted. Ultimately, in the conviction that God abominates the "forcing of conscience," Williams demanded complete freedom of religion and the toleration of even such radical dissenters as the mercilessly castigated Quakers and Anabaptists. (30) Had Williams' ideas gained currency, they must inevitably have toppled the Puritan oligarchy, although Williams himself had no interest in political reform for its own sake. Religious zeal, not humanistic views, led him into collision with the Puritan polity; but once he had blundered into progressive positions, he rarely retreated; and he finally espoused ideals

GO ON TO THE NEXT PAGE

(35) of tolerance and humanity that were not to be realized until many years after his death.

Originally, Williams' tolerance was, rather paradoxically, a function of his Calvinist belief in the total depravity of human nature and the destined damnation of most people. The same pedantic fanaticism which made (40) him object to the name Christendom led him also to object to racial or ethnic discrimination. Since unregenerate "Christians" or those in mortal error such as Roman Catholics were damned no less surely than pagans or Moslems, why prefer one group to another so far as social or civic functions were concerned? And thus, Williams objected to the royal charter also (45) because it failed to acknowledge the land rights of the Indians. He saw government or civil order as merely a convenience for those few elected by God to achieve eternal salvation, and he was accordingly indifferent as to who maintained that order. He even pointed out that unregenerate men could make excellent magistrates.

(50) Williams' real heresy was that he took religious doctrines to their logical conclusions, regardless of the practical consequences.

9. It can be inferred from the passage that Dexter (line 7)

(A) sympathizes with Williams' religious principles while condemning their political consequences
(B) wishes to defend the authorities' expulsion of Williams
(C) views Williams as having been a dangerous fanatic but not a political conspirator
(D) doubts that Williams really was expelled from the colony
(E) considers Williams to have been a troublesome but not malicious man

10. The best title for this passage is

(A) "Roger Williams: the Insolence of Dissent"
(B) "Roger Williams, a Seventeenth-Century Civil Libertarian"
(C) "Roger Williams: an Analysis of a Puritan Heretic"
(D) "Calvinism in the Thought of Roger Williams"
(E) "Roger Williams' Critique of Puritan Society"

11. It can be inferred from the passage that Williams would have been LEAST sympathetic to

(A) an atheist
(B) a political reformer
(C) a royalist
(D) a "visible saint"
(E) an Anabaptist

12. The attitude of the author towards Williams could be best described as

(A) sympathetic and uncritical
(B) objective and critical
(C) ironic and cynical
(D) condescending and approving
(E) biased and defensive

GO ON TO THE NEXT PAGE

13. All of the following can be inferred from the passage EXCEPT

(A) Quakers were not persecuted in the Massachusetts Bay Colony
(B) the king's authority was acknowledged in the Massachusetts Bay Colony
(C) the Massachusetts Bay Colony was not democratic
(D) Williams was a Congregationalist minister
(E) there were inhabitants of the Massachusetts Bay Colony who were not members of the Congregationalist Church

14. On the basis of the passage, it may be inferred that Williams would have been most likely to support

(A) an argument for egalitarianism based on the premise that the Creator has endowed all men equally
(B) a proposal to compel all inhabitants of the Massachusetts Bay Colony to swear allegiance to the civil authorities
(C) a demand for a more democratic method in the selection of magistrates
(D) a proposal to make membership in the Congregationalist Church less exclusive
(E) the appointment of a distinguished Jewish colonel to organize the colonial militia

15. In the light of the passage, an "unregenerate" man (line 20) would best be described as

(A) a religious dissenter
(B) a man rejected on moral grounds from holding public office
(C) a sinner holding church membership
(D) a non-Christian
(E) a man who has not been reborn spiritually

16. In line 25, the phrase "visible saints" is set off by quotation marks primarily in order to

(A) show that the phrase is not to be taken literally
(B) underscore the hypocrisy of Puritan society
(C) indicate that this phrase was used by Williams and his contemporaries
(D) indicate that this is a phrase commonly used by historians specializing in the Puritan period
(E) emphasize the virtuousness required of magistrates

17. It can be inferred from the passage that Williams most directly threatened the Puritan oligarchy in that his

(A) insistence on the total depravity of human nature tarnished the ruling class's image
(B) opposition to the administration of oaths interfered with both judicial and executive processes
(C) toleration of dissenters ran counter to the basis of the Puritan polity
(D) demand that persons not church members be admitted to the magistracy might break the Congregationalist monopoly of government
(E) subordination of civil government to religious doctrine subverted the magistrates' authority

GO ON TO THE NEXT PAGE

Classic economic theory holds that any effort is to be accounted industrial only so far as its ultimate purpose is the utilization of non-human things. The coercive utilization of man by man is not felt to be an industrial function; but all effort directed to enhance human life by
(5) taking advantage of the non-human environment is classed together as industrial activity. Economists in this classic tradition postulate man's "power over nature" as the characteristic fact of industrial productivity. This industrial power over nature is taken to include man's power over the life of animals and over all the elemental forces. A line is drawn in this
(10) way between mankind and brute creation.

However, in primitive societies this line is drawn in a different place and in another way. In such societies and cultures there is an alert and pervading sense of antithesis between two comprehensive groups of phenomena, in one of which primitive man includes himself, and in the other, his
(15) victual. There is a felt antithesis between economic and non-economic phenomena, but it is not conceived in the "civilized" fashion; it lies not between man and brute creation, but between animate and inert things. Of course, in this context the word animate is not equivalent in meaning to the word living. In the primitive frame of reference, the term animate is not
(20) applicable to all living things, and it is applicable to a great many others. Such a striking natural phenomenon as a storm, a disease, or a waterfall is recognized as "animate," while fruits and herbs, and even inconspicuous animals, such as house-flies, maggots, lemmings, and sheep, are not ordinarily apprehended as "animate" except when taken collectively.
(25) To the primitive mind, the elaboration and utilization of what is afforded by inert nature is activity on quite a different plane from dealings with "animate" things and forces. The line of demarcation may be vague and shifting, but the broad distinction is sufficiently real and cogent to influence the primitive scheme of life. To the class of things
(30) apprehended as animate is imputed an unfolding of activity directed to some end. It is this teleological unfolding of activity that constitutes any object or phenomenon an "animate" fact. Wherever the member of a primitive society meets with activity that is at all obtrusive, he construes it in the only terms that are ready to hand — the terms immediately given in his
(35) consciousness of his own actions. Activity is, therefore, assimilated to the human agent. Phenomena of this character — especially those whose behavior is notably formidable or baffling — have to be met in a different spirit and with proficiency of a different kind from that required in dealing with inert things. To deal successfully with such phenomena is a
(40) work of exploit rather than of industry. It is an assertion of prowess, not of diligence.

Under the guidance of this naive discrimination between the inert and the inanimate, the activities of the primitive social group tend to fall into two classes, which we may call exploit and industry. Industry is effort
(45) that goes to create a new thing, with a new purpose given it by the fashioning hand of its maker out of passive ("brute") material, while exploit, so far as it results in an outcome useful to the agent, is the conversion to his own ends of energies previously directed to some other end by another agent. We still speak of "brute matter" with something of the
(50) primitive realization of a profound significance in the term.

GO ON TO THE NEXT PAGE

18. The primary purpose of this passage is to

(A) explain the conception of economic and industrial activities that prevails in primitive societies
(B) trace the origin of the classic economic conception of industrial activity
(C) compare and contrast the classic economic conception of industrial activity with the primitive conception
(D) demonstrate that the primitive distinction between economic and non-economic activity is based on irrationality and logical fallacies
(E) argue that the primitive conception of economic activity is just as logical as the "civilized" conception

19. According to the passage, what is the primary distinction between the classic economic conception of industrial activity and the primitive conception?

(A) While warfare and enslavement are considered "industrial" in the primitive scheme, the exploitation of man by man is not considered "industrial" in classic economic theory.
(B) Classic economic theory does not distinguish between "exploit" and "industry," but this distinction is central in the primitive scheme.
(C) In the classic economic conception, the enhancement of human life by exploitation of the non-human environment is central, whereas in the primitive scheme such enhancement is confined to the utilization of "animate" things.
(D) While classic economic theory sees "man's power over nature" as the main factor in industrial activity, in the primitive scheme the main factor is man's power over "inert" things.
(E) Underlying the primitive conception of industrial activity is an antithesis between animate and inanimate nature, whereas the classic economic conception of industrial activity presupposes an antithesis between man and nature.

20. It may be inferred from the passage that in a primitive community all of the following would be considered acts of exploit EXCEPT

(A) hunting big game
(B) harvesting a field of grain
(C) curing a sick child
(D) raiding a neighboring village
(E) expelling a sorcerer

21. In line 35, the phrase <u>assimilated to</u> most nearly means

(A) likened to
(B) contrasted to
(C) combined with
(D) adapted to
(E) understood as

GO ON TO THE NEXT PAGE

22. According to the passage, which of the following ideas are characteristic of primitive patterns of thought?

I. Animate things are, by definition, those exhibiting life, feeling, and movement.

II. Man is to be sharply distinguished from his food.

III. Storms, floods, and plagues are not random occurrences.

IV. A person's death is always the result of some being's intention.

(A) I, II, III, and IV
(B) II, III, and IV only
(C) I, II, and III only
(D) III and IV only
(E) II and III only

23. All of the following statements are supported by the passage EXCEPT

(A) Members of a primitive society distinguish vaguely but emphatically between animate phenomena and inert phenomena.
(B) A member of a primitive society sees a reflection of human sentience and volition in animate phenomena.
(C) Members of a primitive society conceive of industrial activity as something concerned with inert nature.
(D) The primitive social group values industry less than exploit.
(E) Members of a primitive society consider diligence a primary industrial virtue.

24. The author's diction and usage could best be described as

(A) specialized and technical
(B) formal and literary
(C) colloquial and non-technical
(D) euphemistic and hyperbolic
(E) archaic and outmoded

25. It may be inferred from the final sentence of the passage that the author

(A) finds language occasionally deceptive
(B) sees a parallel between modern and primitive economic conceptions
(C) finds primitive vestiges in modern habits of thought
(D) believes that certain primitive conceptions exhibit profound insight
(E) finds a primitive antithesis between literal and figurative meaning in modern language usage

STOP

YOU MAY CHECK YOUR WORK ON THIS SECTION ONLY UNTIL YOUR TIME IS UP.
DO NOT WORK ON ANY OTHER SECTION.

SECTION II

Time - 30 minutes

20 Questions

Directions: In this section solve each problem, using any available space on the page for scratchwork. Then indicate the best answer of the answer choices given.

Numbers: All numbers used are real numbers.

Figures: Figures that accompany problems in this text are intended to provide information useful in solving the problem. They are drawn as accurately as possible EXCEPT when it is stated in a specific problem that its figure is not drawn to scale. All figures lie in a plane unless otherwise indicated.

1. $\dfrac{1}{\frac{1}{3}+\frac{1}{4}} =$

(A) $\frac{1}{7}$ (B) $\frac{3}{4}$ (C) $\frac{12}{7}$ (D) $\frac{7}{2}$ (E) 7

2. If $4x-1 = 0$ and $xy = 2$, then $y =$

(A) -2 (B) $-\frac{1}{4}$ (C) 2 (D) 4 (E) 8

3. A total of $30,000 invested in two investments yields $4\frac{1}{2}$% and 6% simple interest. If the total interest at the end of the year was $1,470, how much was invested at the higher rate?

(A) $ 8,000
(B) $14,000
(C) $17,500
(D) $22,000
(E) $25,650

4. In country X, a decrease in the average Currency Exchange Rate (CER) of 2% or an increase of the Average Mortgage Rate (AMR) of 1% is reflected as a 10-point increase in the National Retail Price Index. During one month, both the CER and the AMR increased by 1%. What would be the expected change in the National Retail Price Index?

(A) -5 (B) 0 (C) +5 (D) +10 (E) +15

5. For a school sports event, adult tickets cost $3 each and children's tickets cost $1 each. If there were 50 fewer children than adults at the event and the total receipts were $1,110, how many adult tickets were sold?

(A) 165 (B) 260 (C) 265

(D) 290 (E) 310

GO ON TO THE NEXT PAGE

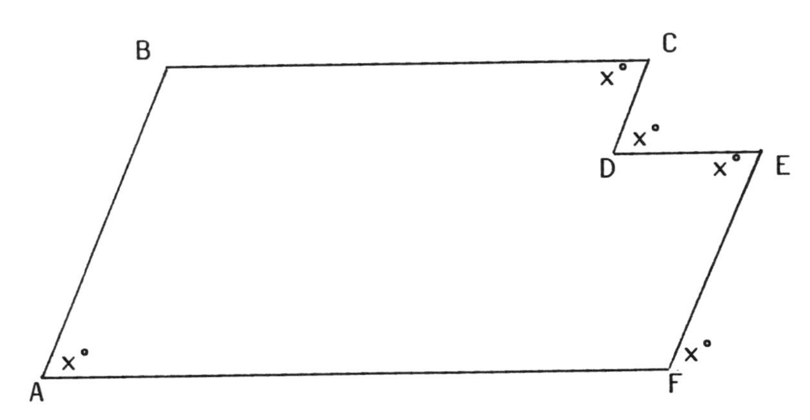

6. In the figure above, BC and AF are 20 centimeters apart while DE and AF are 15 centimeters apart. If the lengths of BC and AF are 30 and 40 centimeters, respectively, and all acute angles = x° as shown, what is the area of the figure in square centimeters?

   (A) 800 (B) 750 (C) 700

   (C) 600 (E) 450

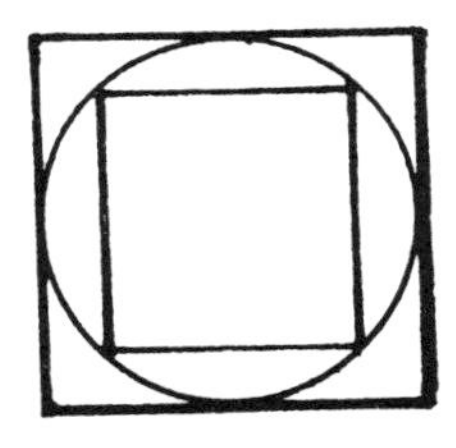

7. For the figure above, what is the ratio of area of the larger square to that of the smaller square?

   (A) $\frac{1}{2\sqrt{2}}$ (B) $\frac{1}{\sqrt{2}}$ (C) $\frac{4}{3}$ (D) $\frac{\sqrt{2}}{1}$ (E) $\frac{2}{1}$

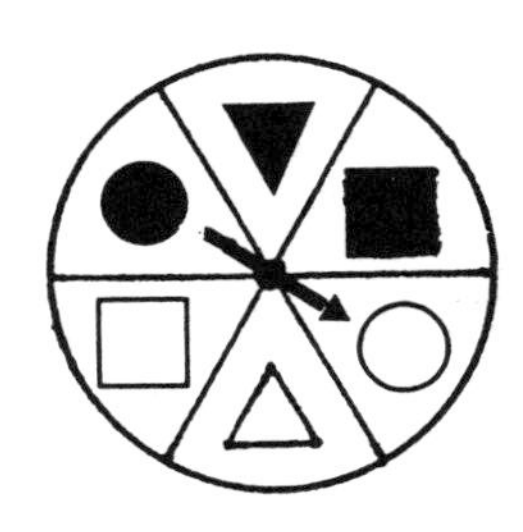

8. The figure above is divided into 6 equal sectors and has a spinner in the form of an arrow pivoted about the center of the figure. If the spinner is rotated 4,140° clockwise from the position shown, towards which symbol will the arrow head point?

   (A) white triangle
   (B) white square
   (C) black circle
   (D) black triangle
   (E) black square

9. A candy mixture to be sold at $1 a pound is to be made from two kinds of candy, one kind that sells at $2 for 3 pounds and a second kind that sells at $3 for 2 pounds. If 60 pounds of the mixture is to be made, how many pounds of the more expensive mixture is to be used?

   (A) 20 (B) 24 (C) 30 (D) 36 (E) 48

10. If R and S are prime numbers, then the product of R and S could be any of the following EXCEPT

    (A) an odd integer
    (B) an even integer
    (C) a divisor of 35
    (D) equal to 30
    (E) less than 10

GO ON TO THE NEXT PAGE

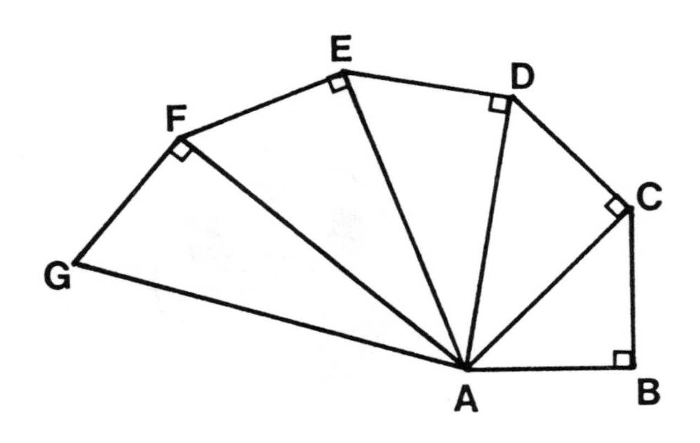

11. For the figure above, AB, BC, CD, DE, EF, and FG are each of length 1. How long is AG?

(A) $\sqrt{3}$
(B) 2
(C) $\sqrt{6}$
(D) $2\sqrt{2}$
(E) $2\sqrt{3}$

12. A six-month $16,000 Certificate of Deposit earns simple interest at the rate of $5\frac{1}{2}$% per annum. What is the total value of the Certificate at the end of six months?

(A) $16,880.00
(B) $16,452.10
(C) $16,440.00
(D) $16,232.10
(E) $16,220.00

13. If $\frac{x}{y} = 2$, then $\frac{xy - x^2}{x^2} =$

(A) $-\frac{1}{2}$ (B) 0 (C) $\frac{1}{2}$ (D) 1 (E) 2

14. In a certain country, the market value of a house can be expected to double every 8 years. A house originally purchased for $8,000 in 1958 would most likely have a market value in 1990 of

(A) $24,000
(B) $32,000
(C) $64,256
(D) $128,000
(E) $256,000

15. John can finish a type of job in 9 days by himself but if he works with Paul, they can do the job in 6 days. If Paul works on this kind of job by himself, how long would it take him to complete it?

(A) 18 (B) 15 (C) 9 (D) 8 (E) $4\frac{1}{2}$

GO ON TO THE NEXT PAGE

16. If M and N are integers such that $-6 < M < 7$ and $-5 < N < 12$, what is the greatest value of

$$M^2 - MN \ ?$$

(A) -40 (B) 0 (C) 25 (D) 60 (E) 80

17. During a four-day sale, a store sells 20% of its stock of kitchen tables on the first day, 25% of the remaining stock on the second day, one-third of the unsold tables on the third day and 50% of what was left on the last day. If 18 tables remained after the sale was over, how many tables were in stock at the beginning of the sale?

(A) 1800 (B) 240 (C) 146 (D) 120 (E) 90

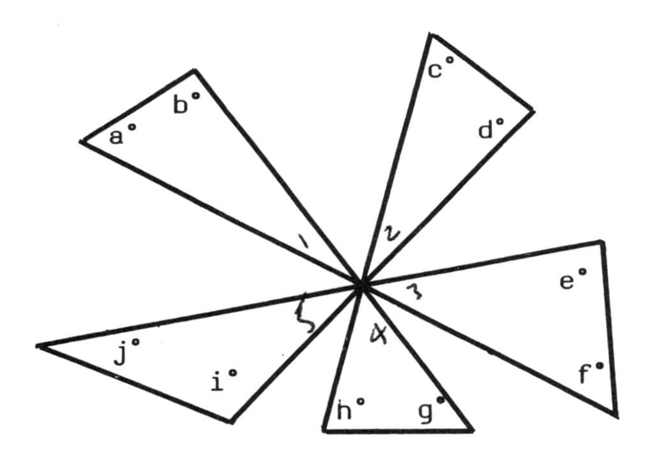

18. In the figure above, 5 triangles are formed by connecting the ends of 5 straight lines through a common point as shown. What is the average (arithmetic mean) of <u>all</u> of the labeled angles, a°, b°, c°, etc., shown above?

(A) 72° (B) 60° (C) 45° (D) 30° (E) 18°

19. During a boat race, the wind pattern forces a sailboat to sail 500 meters due East from point A in order to reach point B, then to sail 600 meters due North to point C, and then 300 meters due East to reach a buoy at point D. After sailing around the buoy, the boat sails in a straight line from D to A. How far, in meters, did the boat sail during the race?

(A) 1500
(B) 2000
(C) 2200
(D) 2400
(E) 2800

20. Which of the following numbers is divisible by 6 but is not divisible by 4 ?

(A) 98765
(B) 987654
(C) 9876543
(D) 98765432
(E) 987654321

S T O P

YOU MAY CHECK YOUR WORK ON THIS SECTION ONLY UNTIL YOUR TIME IS UP.
DO NOT WORK ON ANY OTHER SECTION.

Section III

Time - 30 minutes

25 Questions

Directions: Each passage in this group is followed by questions on content. After reading a passage, choose the best answer to each question and blacken the corresponding space on the answer sheet. Answer all questions following a passage on the basis of what is stated or implied in that passage.

Even in the earlier part of the modern period, English law was not free from caste distinctions. The benefit of clergy, which had originally been an immunity claimed by ecclesiastics from the secular courts, had been gradually transformed into a mere class privilege, whereby educated persons (5) could escape punishment for secondary offenses. Thus in the seventeenth century the question whether a man would be hanged for larceny or not depended on whether he could read, unless indeed he had forfeited the benefit of clergy by contracting a second marriage or by marrying a widow. In 1705 the necessity for reading was abolished, and benefit of clergy could (10) thereafter be claimed by all persons alike for a first offense in the case of secondary crimes. But important distinctions were still made. The offender, unless he was a peer or a clerk in orders, was, until 1779, branded in the hand and liable to seven years' transportation. Clerks in orders, on the other hand, might plead their clergy for any number of (15) offenses, and peers had received the same privileges as clerks by the statute of 1547. However, during the eighteenth century benefit of clergy was gradually withdrawn from an increasing number of offenses; but it was not until 1827 that it was finally abolished, and even then it was doubtful whether the privilege of peers fell with it. This question was not settled (20) until 1841, when the statute of Edward VI was repealed, and peers accused of felony became liable to the same punishments as other persons.

When it is remembered, moreover, that the whole administration of petty justice and of the preliminary process in graver crimes was in the hands of the landed gentry, upon whose estates the laboring classes, rendered (25) landless by economic changes, were fixed by the Act of Settlement (1701), when it is also borne in mind that the same justices had the power of fixing wages, and that the whole of the working classes in the country were always upon or over the verge of pauperism and dependent upon the support of the Poor Law, the control of which was substantially in the same hands, it will (30) be recognized that the nominal freedom of the English laborer down to the beginning of the nineteenth-century reform period was a blessing very much disguised, and that the reality compared unfavorably with the lighter forms of serfdom.

The first stages in the progress of the factory system made matters even (35) worse. The new demand for child labor introduced for a period what was in essence, if not in name, a form of child slavery, pauper children being regularly imported in the manufacturing districts as apprentices and set to work under conditions as to hours and also as to housing which would have been onerous even at less tender years. But these abuses, when fully (40) realized by the public, led with remarkable speed to a series of legislative measures which overrode the so-called freedom of contracts, and protected the children from their legal guardians. The factory system, in short, reproduced the economic conditions under which, in other circumstances, a form of slavery would have arisen. And from this result England and the (45) other industrial nations with it were saved by a distinctively ethical movement.

GO ON TO THE NEXT PAGE

1. Which of the following would be the best title for this passage?

(A) "Benefit of Clergy and Its Legal Consequences"
(B) "The Evolution of Ethics in English Law"
(C) "Social Status and Equality Before the Law in Modern English History"
(D) "Social Injustice in England Prior to the Child Labor Laws"
(E) "Class Privilege in England and the Rise of the Factory System"

2. The presentation in this passage could best be described as

(A) tendentious
(B) ironic
(C) apologetic
(D) detached
(E) ambiguous

3. The author discusses benefit of clergy primarily in order to

(A) compare an inequitable legal institution of medieval origin with early modern inequities
(B) show how existing law could be interpreted to favor persons of superior social status
(C) argue that the basis of English common law was riddled with distinctions of social caste
(D) condemn a significant exception to the uniform application of the criminal code
(E) determine the principle governing the transformation of traditional law into class privilege

4. Which of the following inferences is supported by the passage?

(A) Before 1705 a defendant charged with larceny could escape prosecution by proving his literacy.
(B) A seventeenth-century English clergyman's legal immunity was affected by his wife's marital history.
(C) Before 1827 a peer charged with even a third offense of larceny could claim an immunity analogous to benefit of clergy.
(D) In the seventeenth and eighteenth centuries, women defendants were excluded from benefit of clergy.
(E) Between 1705 and 1779, illiterates, clergymen, and peers enjoyed equal immunity only for a first offense in the case of secondary crimes.

5. In the context in which it appears, the phrase "a blessing very much disguised" (lines 31-32) means most nearly

(A) a curse
(B) a severe disadvantage
(C) one step on a long road
(D) a reduction
(E) an illusion

GO ON TO THE NEXT PAGE

6. The passage contains information to answer which of the following questions?

I. Why was benefit of clergy abolished?

II. What were some of the economic controls upon the English working class?

III. What were some of the legislative measures which corrected the abuses of the factory system?

IV. What effect did the Act of Settlement have?

(A) I, II, and III only
(B) II, III, and IV only
(C) I, III, and IV only
(D) II and IV only
(E) II only

7. It may be inferred from the passage that the author would probably agree with all of the following EXCEPT that

(A) eighteenth-century English justices used the law as a means of keeping the lower classes in their places
(B) some feudal peasants were better off than eighteenth-century English laborers
(C) the abuses of the early factory system were soon corrected by a regulatory mechanism inherent in the system itself
(D) even after 1705 the law relating to benefit of clergy reflected class distinctions
(E) in the seventeenth and eighteenth centuries, literacy was an effective indicator of caste

8. On the basis of the passage, it may be inferred that the objection to the industrial exploitation of children in the early nineteenth century was primarily

(A) political
(B) social
(C) economic
(D) legal
(E) moral

One of the most pervasive phenomena of abnormal psychology is the subliminal invasion of consciousness. Typically, the subject does not realize the source of such invasions, and for him or her, therefore, they take the form of inexplicable impulses to act, of obsessive ideas, or even
(5) of hallucinations. The impulses may take the form of "automatic" writing or speech, the meaning of which is often unknown to the subject. Myers gave the name "automatism," sensory or motor, emotional or intellectual, to this whole complex of effects, due to "uprushes" into consciousness of energies originating in the subliminal levels of the mind.

(10) The simplest example of automatism is the phenomenon of post-hypnotic suggestion. We give to a hypnotized subject, sufficiently susceptible, an order to perform some designated act after he wakes from his hypnotic sleep. He will punctually perform this act but without remembering the suggestion

GO ON TO THE NEXT PAGE

that caused it, and he always improvises a pretext for his behavior if the act seems eccentric. We can even cause the subject to have a vision after waking, and the vision will be seen, with no inkling on the subject's part of its source. In the more explicitly pathological context, as Freud had established by 1900, the subliminal consciousness of hysterics reveals to us whole systems of underground life, in the form of painful memories which lead a parasitic existence, buried outside the primary fields of consciousness, and irrupting periodically into the conscious mind, with hallucinations, pains, convulsions, paralyses of feeling and of motion, and the whole syndrome of hysteria. Insofar as we can alter or remove by suggestion these subconscious memories, the patient's symptoms disappear, for such symptoms were automatisms.

(15) (20) (25)

We may conclude that whenever we observe a phenomenon of automatism, whether motor impulse, obsession, eccentricity, delusion, or hallucination, we will find an incursion into ordinary consciousness of ideas elaborated in the subliminal mind. Thus we begin by looking for the source of automatic phenomena in the subconscious life. In hysteria, the lost memories which are the source must be extracted from the patient's unconscious by analysis and other therapy. In psychopathic obsessions or schizophrenic dissociation, the source is more problematic, but by analogy it should also be found in those subliminal regions of the mind first charted by Freud.

(30)

We may further conclude that these subliminal regions accumulate vestiges of perceived experience (whether inattentively or attentively registered) and subconsciously "incubate" motives deposited by a growing sum of experiences. Such motives and ideas are elaborated under such tension that they may enter consciousness with a burst. We may thus interpret all otherwise unaccountable invasive alterations of consciousness as results of subliminal memories reaching the bursting-point.

(35) (40)

9. In this passage the author is primarily concerned with

(A) developing the corollary to a principle
(B) supporting a hypothesis
(C) drawing an analogy
(D) deducing a cause
(E) explaining an effect

10. The author could probably best be described as a

(A) social scientist
(B) psychiatrist
(C) hypnotist
(D) pathologist
(E) historian of psychology

11. Which of the following statements about the phenomenon of post-hypnotic suggestion is supported by the passage?

(A) It is involuntary.
(B) It involves delusion.
(C) It is symptomatic.
(D) It is universal among patients.
(E) It is invariably rationalized by the subject.

GO ON TO THE NEXT PAGE

12. This passage contains information to answer which of the following questions?

I. What is the definition of "automatic" writing?

II. What is autosuggestion?

III. What are the symptoms of hysteria?

(A) I, II, and III
(B) I and II only
(C) I and III only
(D) I only
(E) III only

13. In the context of the passage, the phrase "parasitic existence" (line 20) implies most strongly that

(A) the convulsions and paralyses of hysteria are analogous to those of certain diseases caused by internal parasites
(B) the existence of painful, subliminal memories may be detected only by pathological investigation
(C) the "underground life" of hysterics includes delusions of parasitic infection
(D) subliminal memories prey upon hysterics' conscious minds
(E) the repression of painful memories does not prevent their taking a fearful toll upon the nervous system

14. The author's attitude towards his material could best be described as

(A) complacent
(B) confident
(C) sardonic
(D) hesitant
(E) indifferent

15. It may be inferred from the passage that

(A) repressed memories are the cause of schizophrenic dissociation
(B) the motives behind deviant behavior or eccentricity are created in the subliminal regions of the mind
(C) virtually all mental abnormality may be traced to the phenomenon of automatism
(D) hypnosis has not been successfully used to locate the source of psychopathic obsession
(E) hallucinations are not a form of automatism

16. The passage includes all of the following EXCEPT

(A) refutation
(B) exposition
(C) exemplification
(D) documentation
(E) deduction

GO ON TO THE NEXT PAGE

The standard of reputability requires that dress should show wasteful expenditure, but all wastefulness offends native taste. People instinctively abhor futility of effort or of expenditure, as Nature abhors a vacuum. But the principle of conspicuous waste requires an obviously futile (5) expenditure; and the resulting conspicuous expensiveness of dress is therefore intrinsically ugly. Hence in all innovations in dress, each added or altered detail strives to avoid condemnation by showing some ostensible purpose, while the requirement of conspicuous waste prevents the purposefulness of these innovations from becoming anything more than a (10) transparent pretense. Even at its freest, fashion rarely fails to simulate some ostensible use. The ostensible usefulness of the fashionable details of dress, however, is always so transparent a sham, and their substantial futility presently reveals itself so baldly as to become unbearable, and then we take refuge in a new style. But the new style must conform to the (15) requirement of reputable wastefulness and futility. Its futility presently becomes as odious as its predecessor's; and the only remedy is to seek relief in some new construction, equally futile and untenable. Hence the essential ugliness and unceasing change of fashionable attire.

A new style comes into vogue and remains in favor for a season, and, so (20) long as it is a novelty, it is considered attractive. The prevailing fashion is felt to be beautiful. This is due partly to the relief it affords in being different from what went before it, partly to its being reputable. The canon of reputability partly shapes our tastes; under its guidance anything will be accepted as becoming until its novelty wears off, (25) or until the warrant of reputability is transferred to a new and novel structure. That the alleged beauty of the styles in vogue at any given time is transient and spurious only is attested by the fact that none of the many shifting fashions last. The best fashions of a few years before now seem grotesque or unsightly. Our transient attachment to whatever is the latest (30) rests on other than esthetic grounds, and lasts only until our abiding esthetic sense has had time to assert itself and reject this latest indigestible contrivance.

The process of developing an esthetic nausea takes some time, the length of time required in any given case being in inverse proportion to the (35) degree of intrinsic odiousness of the style in question. This time relation between odiousness and instability in fashions suggests that the more rapidly the styles displace one another, the more offensive they are to sound taste. Therefore, the further the community develops in wealth and mobility, the more imperatively will the law of conspicuous waste assert (40) itself, the more will the sense of beauty tend to atrophy, the more rapidly will the fashions change, and the more grotesque and intolerable will be the styles that successively come into vogue.

17. The author's primary purpose in this passage is to

(A) dispute a commonly accepted position
(B) predict a development
(C) analyze causes and effects
(D) resolve paradoxes
(E) solve a problem

GO ON TO THE NEXT PAGE

18. This passage is most probably an excerpt from

(A) a history of esthetics
(B) an economic analysis of social behavior
(C) a treatise on cultural anthropology
(D) an article on business communications
(E) a book on ethics in life style

19. The author of this passage would be most likely to agree with which of the following statements about fashions in dress?

(A) the degree of revulsion inspired by a dress style is directly related to the futility of that style
(B) the rate of change of fashions varies inversely with the degree of odiousness of the fashions
(C) new styles of dress usually exhibit a plausible usefulness in order to disarm criticism
(D) standards of taste in dress are purely relative
(E) consumers do not generally desire both respectability and utility in dress

20. The author uses a proverbial expression (lines 3-4) primarily in order to

(A) contrast the artificiality of modern fashion with traditional styles
(B) intimate an analogy between the natural sciences and the social sciences
(C) show the natural basis of the principle of conspicuous waste
(D) suggest a metaphoric vacuum in modern culture
(E) emphasize man's innate detestation of waste

21. According to the author, new fashions in dress are characterized by all of the following EXCEPT

(A) unnecessary expense
(B) make-believe ornamentation
(C) innovation
(D) an attempt to disarm criticism
(E) factitious utility

22. The word spurious (line 27) means most nearly

(A) ostensible
(B) untenable
(C) homologous
(D) false
(E) temporary

GO ON TO THE NEXT PAGE

23. The tone of this passage could best be described as

(A) caustic and ironic
(B) pedantic and hypercritical
(C) bitter and self-righteous
(D) solemn and humorless
(E) plaintive and depressed

24. The author's argument assumes an antithesis between

(A) beauty and taste
(B) novelty and stability
(C) reputability and futility
(D) fashion and utility
(E) usefulness and expensiveness

25. It can be inferred from the passage that a new style of fashionable dress will exhibit

(A) a mimicry of some detail of work clothes
(B) a design using the maximum of expensive material to the least purpose
(C) a feature designed to wear out quickly
(D) deliberately grotesque or unsightly details
(E) a feature designed to malfunction

STOP

YOU MAY CHECK YOUR WORK ON THIS SECTION ONLY UNTIL YOUR TIME IS UP.
DO NOT WORK ON ANY OTHER SECTION.

SECTION IV

Time - 30 minutes

25 Questions

Directions: Each of the data sufficiency problems below consists of a question and two statements, labeled (1) and (2), in which certain data are given. You have to decide whether the data given in the statements are sufficient for answering the question. Using the data given in the statements plus your knowledge of mathematics and everyday facts (such as the number of days in July or the meaning of counterclockwise), you are to blacken space

- A if statement (1) ALONE is sufficient, but statement (2) alone is not sufficient to answer the question asked;
- B if statement (2) ALONE is sufficient, but statement (1) alone is not sufficient to answer the question asked;
- C if BOTH statements (1) and (2) TOGETHER are sufficient to answer the question asked, but NEITHER statement ALONE is sufficient;
- D if EACH statement ALONE is sufficient to answer the question asked;
- E if statements (1) and (2) TOGETHER are NOT sufficient to answer the question asked, and additional data specific to the problem are needed.

Numbers: All numbers used are real numbers.

Figures: A figure in a data sufficiency problem will conform to the information given in the question, but will not necessarily conform to the additional information given in statements (1) and (2).

You may assume that lines shown as straight are straight and that angle measures are greater than zero.

You may assume that the position of points, angles, regions, etc., exist in the order shown.

All figures lie in a plane unless otherwise indicated.

Examples:

In triangle PQR, what is the value of x?

(1) PQ = PR

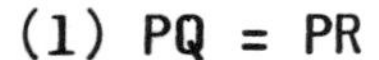

(2) y = 40

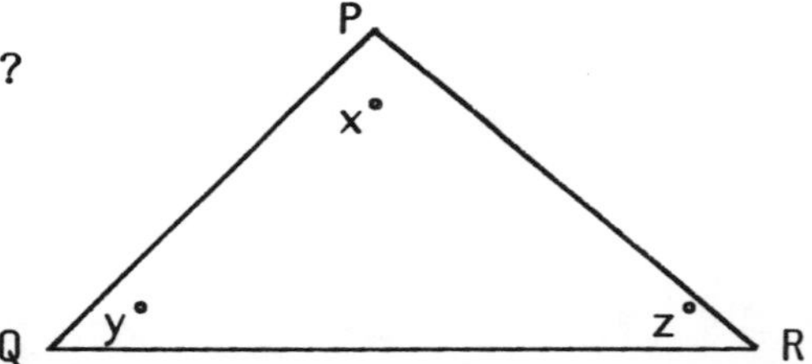

Explanation: According to statement (1), PQ = PR; therefore, triangle PQR is isosceles and y = z. Since x+y+z = 180, x+2y = 180. Since statement (1) does not give a value for y, you cannot answer the question using statement (1) by itself. According to statement (2), y = 40; therefore, x+z = 140. Since statement (2) does not give a value for z, you cannot answer the question using statement (2) by itself. Using both statements together, you can find y and z; therefore, you can find x, and the answer to the problem is C.

GO ON TO THE NEXT PAGE

A Statement (1) ALONE is sufficient, but statement (2) alone is not sufficient.
B Statement (2) ALONE is sufficient, but statement (1) alone is not sufficient.
C BOTH statements TOGETHER are sufficient, but NEITHER statement alone is sufficient.
D EACH statement ALONE is sufficient.
E Statements (1) and (2) TOGETHER are NOT sufficient.

1. A 300-centimeter-long shelf is to be cut into 4 pieces. If the 2 middle-sized pieces are the same size, how big is the longest piece?

   (1) The combined length of 2 pieces is 130 centimeters.

   (2) The shortest piece is exactly 60 centimeters long.

2. In a supermarket, $2,000 worth of brand X soda was sold by the case in June. What was the value of the cases of brand X soda sold in July?

   (1) During July, cases of brand X were reduced 10% in price.

   (2) There were 22% more cases of brand X sold in July than were sold in June.

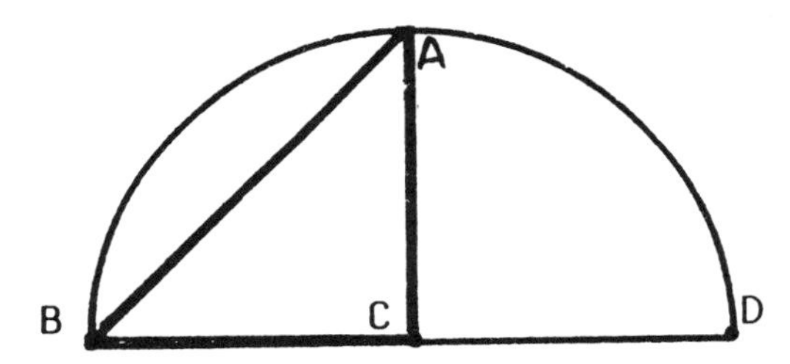

3. In the figure above, angle ABC is 45°. If C is the center of the semi-circle, what is the area of the triangle ABC?

   (1) The length of arc AB is 2π.

   (2) BD = 8

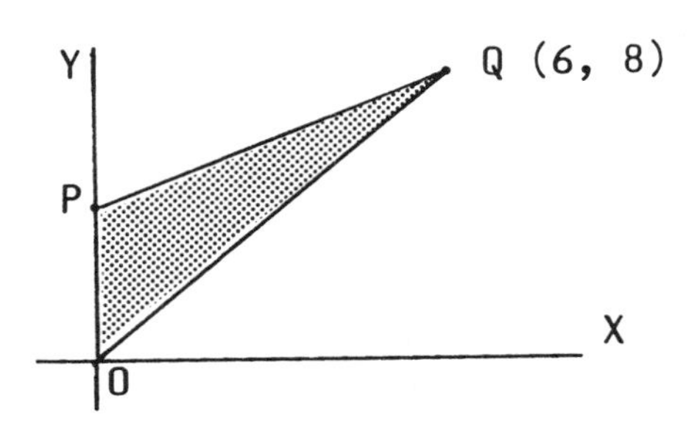

4. What is the area of the shaded region shown above?

   (1) P has coordinates, (0, 5).

   (2) OQ = 10

5. A swimming pool was filled to capacity by 3 intake pipes. What percent of the volume was filled by the pipe with the lowest flow rate?

   (1) The pipes flowed continuously for 4 hours at the rate of 20, 40, and 50 gallons of water per minute, respectively.

   (2) The largest pipe supplied water at 2.5 times the rate of the smallest pipe.

GO ON TO THE NEXT PAGE

A Statement (1) ALONE is sufficient, but statement (2) alone is not sufficient.
B Statement (2) ALONE is sufficient, but statement (1) alone is not sufficient.
C BOTH statements TOGETHER are sufficient, but NEITHER statement alone is sufficient.
D EACH statement ALONE is sufficient.
E Statements (1) and (2) TOGETHER are NOT sufficient.

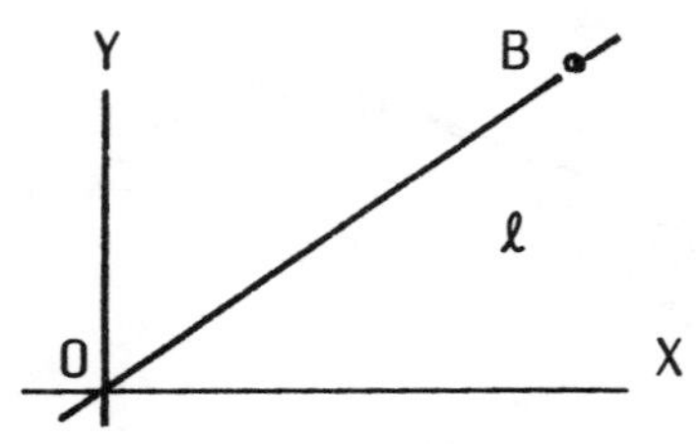

6. Is $y = x$ the equation of the line ℓ in the figure above?

(1) The angle between the line and the x-axis is 45°.

(2) The point, B, has coordinates, (7, 7).

7. The rectangular floor plan for a new house was changed to a square floor plan. If one dimension was increased 1 meter and the other was decreased 3 meters, what is the area of the new floor plan?

(1) The original length was 4 meters longer than the width.

(2) The original area was 96 square meters.

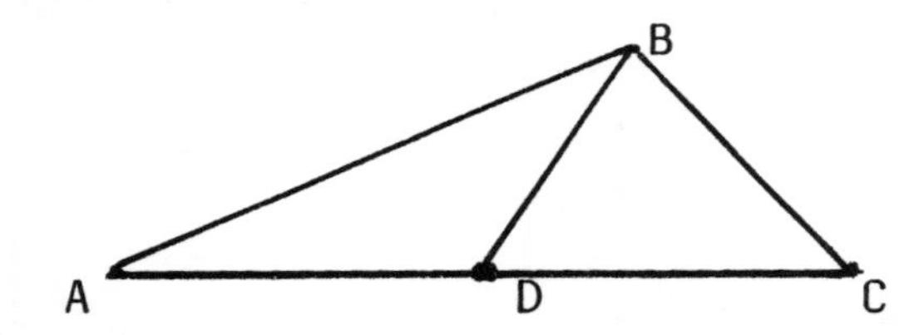

8. What is the area of triangle ABC if CD = 10 ?

(1) The areas of triangles ABD and BDC are equal.

(2) BD is perpendicular to AD.

9. The 3,000 single-crop farmers in Clarke County grow either wheat, oats, or rye. Is wheat grown by most of the single-crop farmers in the county?

(1) There are two single-crop farmers who grow wheat for every one that grows oats.

(1) Of the single-crop farmers in Clarke County, 300 grow rye.

10. Is $x^4 - y^4$ negative?

(1) $0.75 < \frac{x}{y} < 1$

(2) $|x| \neq 1$

GO ON TO THE NEXT PAGE

A Statement (1) ALONE is sufficient, but statement (2) alone is not sufficient.
B Statement (2) ALONE is sufficient, but statement (1) alone is not sufficient.
C BOTH statements TOGETHER are sufficient, but NEITHER statement alone is sufficient.
D EACH statement ALONE is sufficient.
E Statements (1) and (2) TOGETHER are NOT sufficient.

11. Students in a course on Economics were found to read at least one of the three daily newspapers, X, Y, and Z. Of the 30 students, how many read all three newspapers?

(1) Of the 18 who read X, 12 read only X and 4 read just one other newspaper.

(2) Of all the students, 19 read one paper and 9 read just two papers.

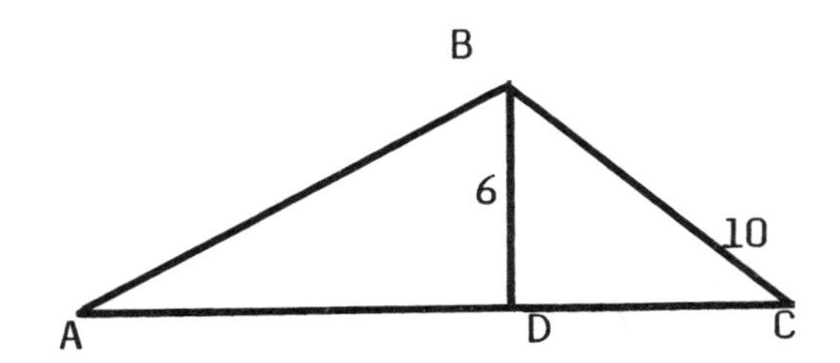

12. In the figure above, what is the length of AB?

(1) AD = 12

(2) Angle BCD = 30°

13. Is the average (arithmetic mean) of five integers greater than 10?

(1) The product of the numbers is 0.

(2) The sum of the numbers is 51.

14. If A, B, C, D, E, ... is a list of all positive prime numbers in ascending order, and N is some positive integer, is $\frac{N}{A}$ an integer?

(1) $\frac{N}{6}$ is an integer.

(2) $\frac{N}{14}$ is an integer.

15. The base alone of a rectangular box has the same area as the <u>total</u> surface area of a cube of side, x. what is the ratio of the volume of the rectangular box to that of the cube?

(1) The longest side of the base of the box is 3 times the length of the side of the cube.

(2) Exactly 18 of the cubes would just fit inside the box.

16. If x is an odd integer, how large is x?

(1) $30.1 < 7x < 48.3$

(2) $\frac{1}{2}x > 2.45$

GO ON TO THE NEXT PAGE

A Statement (1) ALONE is sufficient, but statement (2) alone is not sufficient.
B Statement (2) ALONE is sufficient, but statement (1) alone is not sufficient.
C BOTH statements TOGETHER are sufficient, but NEITHER statement alone is sufficient.
D EACH statement ALONE is sufficient.
E Statements (1) and (2) TOGETHER are NOT sufficient.

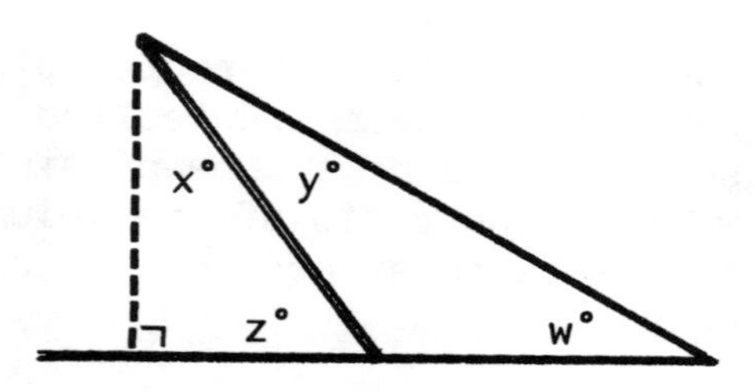

17. In the triangle above, is $x < y$?

(1) $z = 2x$

(2) $w > 2y$

18. If $x \neq 2$, what is the value of

$$\frac{(x-2)^n}{5} + \frac{(2-x)^n}{5} ?$$

(1) $x^3 = 27$

(2) $\frac{1}{2}n$ has a remainder of 1.

19. In the expression, a * (b * c), the symbol * represents which one of the following four mathematical operators, +, −, x, ÷ ?

(1) 1 * (2 * 1) = (1 * 2) * 1

(2) 12 * (1 * 1) = 12

20. A sequence of different numbers beginning with 7 is created by multiplying a preceding number by the positive integer, N. What is the fifth number in the sequence?

(1) The 4th and 5th numbers differ by four times as much as the difference between the 2nd and 3rd numbers.

(2) The product of the 3rd and 4th numbers is 14 times larger than the 5th number.

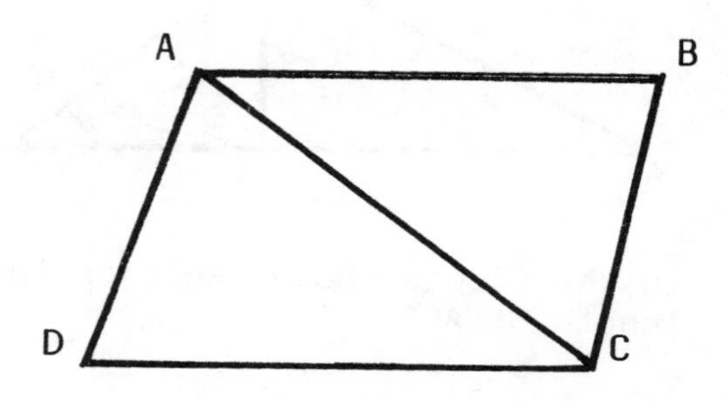

21. In the figure above, AB || DC and angle ABC = 60°. If DC = 12, what is the area of ABCD?

(1) AC divides the figure into two similar triangles and AB = BC.

(2) Angle BAC = angle ACD

GO ON TO THE NEXT PAGE

A Statement (1) ALONE is sufficient, but statement (2) alone is not sufficient.
B Statement (2) ALONE is sufficient, but statement (1) alone is not sufficient.
C BOTH statements TOGETHER are sufficient, but NEITHER statement alone is sufficient.
D EACH statement ALONE is sufficient.
E Statements (1) and (2) TOGETHER are NOT sufficient.

22. If A and B represent non-zero digits in the five-digit number, 12,3AB, is the number 12,3AB divisible by 12?

(1) $A + B = 6$

(2) The three-digit number, 3AB, has a remainder of 4 when divided by 8.

23. Is a 100-meter roll of fencing sufficient to fence in a rectangular garden?

(1) The length of the garden is twice its width.

(2) The garden is 30 meters on one side.

24. If x and y are different positive integers not equal to 3, which is the greater,

$$\frac{x}{y} \quad \text{or} \quad \frac{x+3}{y+3} \quad ?$$

(1) $x < 4$

(2) $y < x$

25. The 95 members of a sports club are to elect a new president from a slate of four candidates, J, K, L, and M. If each member cast just one vote, did M receive the greatest number of votes?

(1) No candidate received as few votes as J, who had 15 votes.

(2) Candidates K and L received 40% of the votes between them.

STOP

YOU MAY CHECK YOUR WORK ON THIS SECTION ONLY UNTIL YOUR TIME IS UP.
DO NOT WORK ON ANY OTHER SECTION.

SECTION V

Time – 30 minutes

20 Questions

Directions: In this section solve each problem, using any available space on the page for scratchwork. Then indicate the best answer of the answer choices given.

Numbers: All numbers used are real numbers.

Figures: Figures that accompany problems in this text are intended to provide information useful in solving the problem. They are drawn as accurately as possible EXCEPT when it is stated in a specific problem that its figure is not drawn to scale. All figures lie in a plane unless otherwise indicated.

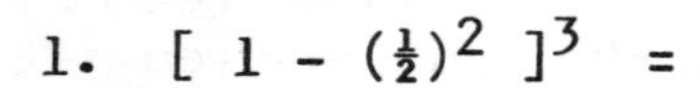

1. $[\,1 - (\frac{1}{2})^2\,]^3 =$

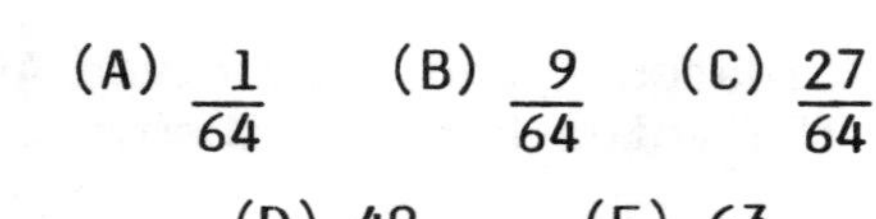

(A) $\frac{1}{64}$ (B) $\frac{9}{64}$ (C) $\frac{27}{64}$ (D) $\frac{49}{64}$ (E) $\frac{63}{64}$

2. A car dealer sold two cars for $4,800 each. If he made a profit of 25% on one of the cars but had a loss of 25% on the other, what was the net gain or loss on both transactions?

(A) $800 loss (B) 0 (C) $800 gain (D) $1,600 (E) none of these

3. A three-digit number is formed from three different digits. A second number is formed by interchanging the first and last digits of the original number. If the second number is subtracted from the first number then the result is always

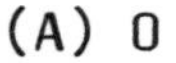

(A) 0
(B) negative
(C) even
(D) a multiple of 6
(E) divisible by 11

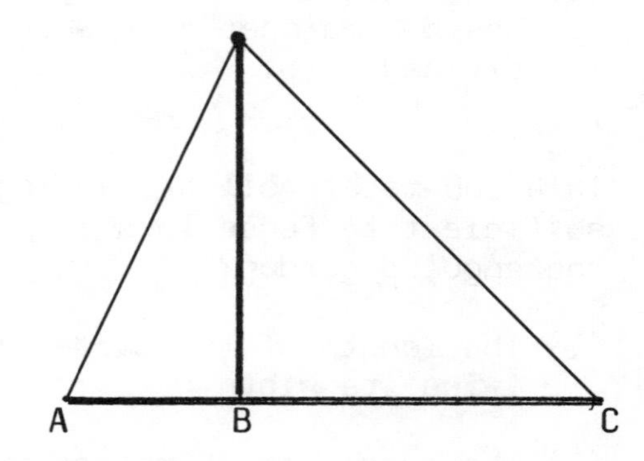

4. A flagpole erected at point B is 12 meters high. Attached to the top of the flagpole are two cables anchored to the ground at points A and C. If the cable lengths are 13 and 15 meters, respectively, and points A, B, and C are in a straight line, how many meters is it from point A to point C ?

(A) 28 (B) 21 (C) 18 (D) 14 (E) 10

GO ON TO THE NEXT PAGE

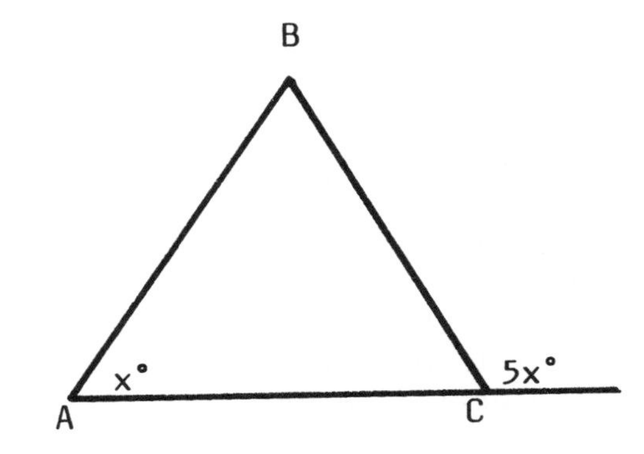

5. In the figure above, AB = BC. If the exterior angle at C is 5x°, what is the value of x?

(A) 150 (B) 120 (C) 90

(D) 60 (E) 30

6. The $\sqrt{2^3 3^3 4^3 6^3}$ equals

(A) $144\sqrt{18}$

(B) $2^2(3)(4)(6)$

(C) $2^2(3)(4)6^2$

(D) $2^2(3)4^2 6^2$

(E) $2^6 3^3 6$

7. $[\sqrt{5} - \sqrt{45}]^2 =$

(A) 20
(B) $\sqrt{50}$
(C) $50 - \sqrt{45}$
(D) - 40
(E) - 1600

8. A racing car driver qualifies for a race by making one circuit of a 10-kilometer track at 120 kph and a second circuit at 200 kph. What is his average speed for the two laps?

(A) 170
(B) 165
(C) 160
(D) 155
(E) 150

9. $\frac{(0.79)^2 - (0.75)^2}{2}$ is approximately

(A) 0.003 (B) $\frac{31}{1000}$ (C) 0.31

(D) 3.1 (E) 31

10. Sequences of numbers can be formed using the rule that each term is one less than twice the previous term. If no two numbers in such sequence may be the same, which of the following numbers <u>cannot</u> be a member of such a sequence?

(A) - 2
(B) - ½
(C) + 1
(D) any prime number
(D) 125

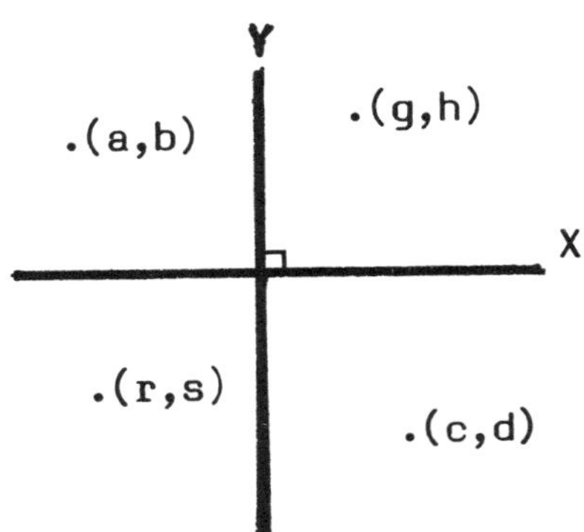

11. In the figure above, all of the relationships below are possible EXCEPT

(A) $r^2 > s$

(B) $r^2 + s^2 > g^2 + h^2$

(C) $ac > bd$

(D) $bd > r^2$

(E) $ad + bd > s^2$

GO ON TO THE NEXT PAGE

12. The value of $\dfrac{60^3}{[(5)(4)(3)(2)(1)]^3}$ is

(A) less than 1
(B) equal to 1
(C) between 1 and 6
(D) equal to 6
(E) greater than 6

13. Sufficient salt was added to 30 kilograms of a 10% salt solution to increase the salt concentration to 25%. How many kilograms of salt were added?

(A) 2
(B) 3
(C) 4
(D) 5
(E) 6

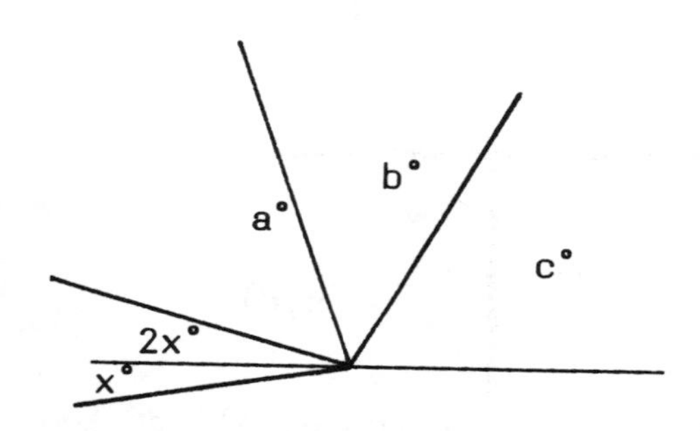

14. In the figure above, each of the angles, a, b, and c equals the sum of the two angles counterclockwise to it, for example,

$$b^\circ = a^\circ + 2x,$$
$$c^\circ = b^\circ + a^\circ.$$

If ABC is a straight line, how big is the largest angle?

(A) 50° (B) 60° (C) 70°
(D) 80° (E) 90°

15. Any number, when divided by 9, has a remainder equal to the sum of its digits. If the last digit of a seven digit number is 4 and the remaining six digits add up to 23, then the original number must be

(A) divisible by 7
(B) divisible by 18
(C) divisible by 23
(D) divisible by 27
(E) a prime number

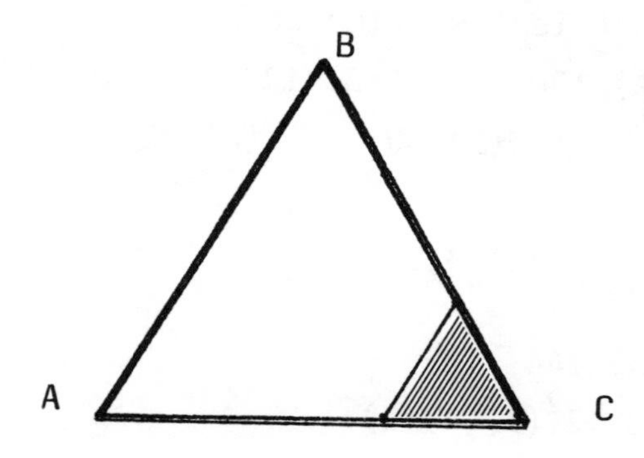

16. In the figure above, the shaded triangle has equal sides of length 1. If AC = BC = 3, what is the area of the unshaded portion of triangle ABC as a fraction of the total area of triangle ABC?

(A) $\frac{8}{9}$ (B) $\frac{7}{8}$ (C) $\frac{2}{3}$
(D) $\frac{3}{8}$ (E) $\frac{1}{9}$

GO ON TO THE NEXT PAGE

17. A car dealer has a large inventory of cars of which 35% are red, 25% are blue, 10% are black and the remainder are other colors. For each color of car, 80% are equipped with automatic transmission and of these, 30% have air-conditioning. What is the probability that a car chosen at random will not be black and will have both automatic transmission and air-conditioning?

(A) $\frac{3}{125}$ (B) $\frac{12}{125}$ (C) $\frac{27}{125}$ (D) $\frac{6}{25}$ (E) $\frac{9}{10}$

18. A 4,000 liter tank, half-full of water is being filled from a pipe with a flow rate of 1 kiloliter every 2 minutes. At the same time, the tank is losing water from two drains at the rate of 1 kiloliter every 4 minutes and 1 kiloliter every 6 minutes. How many minutes does it take to fill the tank completely?

(A) 8 (B) 12 (C) 18 (D) 24 (E) 48

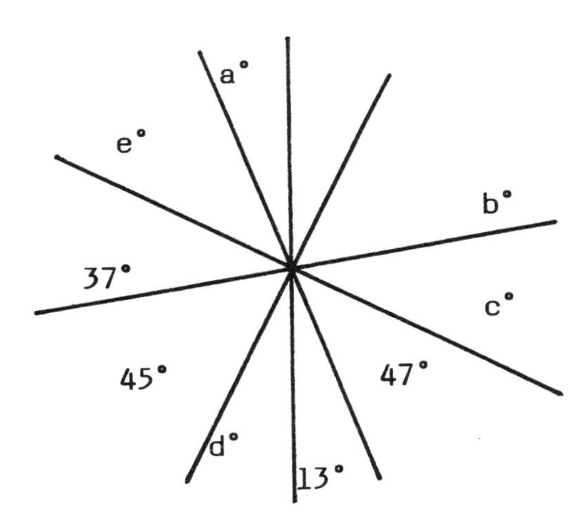

19. In the figure above, a + b + c + d equals

(A) 133 (B) 120 (C) 97 (D) 82 (E) 50

20. A nature preserve is located on a rectangular piece of land. If one side is 6 kilometers long and a straight, $6\frac{1}{2}$-kilometer-path runs diagonally from one corner to the corner opposite, what is the area of the land in square kilometers?

(A) 48
(B) 39
(C) 24
(D) $19\frac{1}{2}$
(E) 15

STOP

YOU MAY CHECK YOUR WORK ON THIS SECTION ONLY UNTIL YOUR TIME IS UP.
DO NOT WORK ON ANY OTHER SECTION.

SECTION VI

Time: 30 minutes

25 Questions

Directions: In each of the following sentences, some part of the sentence or the entire sentence is underlined. Beneath each sentence you will find five ways of phrasing the underlined part. The first of these repeats the original; the other four are different. If you think the original is better than any of the alternatives, choose answer A; otherwise choose one of the others. Select the best version and blacken the corresponding space on your answer sheet.

This is a test of correctness and effectiveness of expression. In choosing answers, follow the requirements of standard written English; that is, pay attention to grammar, choice of words, and sentence construction. Choose the answer that expresses most effectively what is presented in the original sentence; this answer should be clear and exact, without awkwardness, ambiguity, or redundancy.

1. Two types of consumer, one associated with a middle-class life style and the other less easily linked to any class, responds to such an appeal and contributes to the strength of the market.

   (A) responds to such an appeal and contributes
   (B) respond to such an appeal and contributing
   (C) respond to such an appeal and contribute
   (D) respond to such an appeal and contributes
   (E) responding to such an appeal, contributes

2. In her powerful novel "Wuthering Heights," Emily Brontë portrays, in Heathcliff, one of the most titanic characters in literature.

   (A) her powerful novel "Wuthering Heights," Emily Brontë portrays
   (B) Emily Brontë's powerful novel "Wuthering Heights," the author portrays
   (C) Emily Brontë's powerful novel "Wuthering Heights" is portrayed
   (D) Emily Brontë's powerful novel "Wuthering Heights," she portrays
   (E) the powerful novel "Wuthering Heights" by Emily Brontë, the authoress portrays

3. Until his battle fleet and transports were destroyed by the Royal Navy, Napoleon had been intending the invasion of Britain.

   (A) had been intending the invasion of
   (B) was intending the invasion of
   (C) had intended invading
   (D) had intended to invade
   (E) intended invading

GO ON TO THE NEXT PAGE

4. He is now the only member of the school board who is opposed to Ms. Martinez getting the post of senior high school principal, though they had previously been equally divided over the appointment.

(A) is opposed to Ms. Martinez
(B) is opposed to Ms. Martinez'
(C) are opposed to Ms. Martinez
(D) is opposing to Ms. Martinez'
(E) are opposed to Ms. Martinez'

5. The building commission specified that the structures must be rectangular, with a length of twenty meters, a width of ten meters, and a height of seven meters, as recommended by the architect.

(A) rectangular, with a length of twenty meters, a width of ten meters, and a height of seven meters,
(B) rectangular in shape, with a length of twenty meters, a width of ten meters, and seven meters high
(C) rectangular in shape, twenty meters long by ten meters wide, and seven meters high
(D) rectangular as to shape, with a twenty-meter length, a ten-meter width, and a seven-meter height
(E) rectangular, having a twenty meters length, a ten meters width, and a seven meters height

6. Of the various mammalian groups included in the arboreal fauna of the eastern region, the lemur is the largest, and it is among the few primate genera that forage nocturnally.

(A) largest, and it is among the few primate genera that forage
(B) largest, and it is among the few primate genera that forages
(C) larger, and it is among the few primate genera that forages
(D) larger, and it is among the few primate genera that forage
(E) larger, and it is among the few primate genera foraging

7. The Pilgrim Fathers of Plymouth Colony had originally emigrated from England in search of freedom to practice their brand of Puritanism; they severely punished religious dissenters in their own colony.

(A) The Pilgrim Fathers of Plymouth Colony had originally emigrated from England in search of freedom to practice their brand of Puritanism;
(B) Although the Pilgrim Fathers of Plymouth Colony had originally emigrated from England in search of freedom to practice their brand of Puritanism,
(C) While the Pilgrim Fathers of Plymouth Colony originally emigrated from England in search of freedom to practice their brand of Puritanism,
(D) The Pilgrim Fathers of Plymouth Colony originally emigrated from England in search of freedom to practice their brand of Puritanism, but
(E) The Pilgrim Fathers of Plymouth Colony had originally emigrated from England in search of freedom to practice their brand of Puritanism, and

GO ON TO THE NEXT PAGE

8. The weight of an adult male kodiak bear, the largest of all quadruped carnivores, is greater than those of two lions' combined.

(A) those of two lions'
(B) that of two lions' weights
(C) two lions weights
(D) that of two lions
(E) two lions

9. A bachelor's degree from Central University not only carries the prestige of a high-quality education but it also assures that the student has been excellently prepared for either graduate study, professional training, or career entry.

(A) not only carries the prestige of a high-quality but it also assures that the student
(B) carries not only the prestige of a high-quality education but also the assurance that the holder of that degree
(C) carries not only the prestige of a high-quality education but it also ensures that the student
(D) not only carries the prestige of a high-quality education but also the assurance that the holder of that degree
(E) carries not only the prestige of a high-quality education; it also assures that the student

10. In response to the sales manager's suggestion, the chairperson indicated that the export market, due to the enterprise of several competitors, was already filled.

(A) export market, due to the enterprise of several competitors, was already filled
(B) filling of the export market was already due to the enterprise of several competitors
(C) export market, consequent on several competitors' enterprise, was already filled
(D) export market was already filled due to the enterprise of several competitors
(E) export market was already filled as a result of the enterprise of several competitors

11. Staff Sergeant Angelina King was responsible for the reception of the women trainees, their initial issuance of linen, blankets, and fatigues, and their assignment to barracks.

(A) their assignment
(B) the assignment of them
(C) assigning them
(D) the assigning of them
(E) their assigning

GO ON TO THE NEXT PAGE

12. Each of these sixteenth-century physicists persisted in their demonstration that the earth is round, despite their fear of the Inquisition.

(A) their demonstration that the earth is round, despite their
(B) his demonstration that the earth is round, despite his
(C) his demonstration that the earth is round, despite their
(D) their demonstration that the earth was round, despite their
(E) his demonstration that the earth was round, despite his

13. Responding to the need for better information control within industry, managers' interest in computer networking has grown steadily throughout the past three years.

(A) managers' interest in computer networking has grown steadily
(B) the interest of managers in computer networking has grown steadily
(C) managers' interest in computer networking grew steadily
(D) managers have shown a steadily growing interest in computer networking
(E) managers showed a steadily growing interest in computer networking

14. Science teachers should ensure that students have a thorough grasp of facts, natural laws, and accepted theories; but, ideally, creative thinking and new approaches to old problems should also be promoted.

(A) theories; but, ideally, creative thinking and new approaches to old problems should also be promoted
(B) theories, but it would be ideal if creative thinking and new approaches to old problems should also be promoted by them
(C) theories, but, ideally, also promoting creative thinking and new approaches to old problems
(D) theories, but promoting creative thinking and new approaches to old problems should, ideally, also be done
(E) theories; but, ideally, they should also promote creative thinking and new approaches to old problems

15. Increased deregulation in industries ranging from ship-building to cosmetics has combined with shifts in the demarcation of the public sector to alter almost radically the business climate and make nonsense of economic prognostications.

(A) has combined with shifts in the demarcation of the public sector to alter almost radically
(B) has combined with shifts in the demarcation of the public sector to almost alter radically
(C) have combined with shifts in the demarcation of the public sector almost radically to alter
(D) have combined with shifts in the demarcation of the public sector to alter almost radically
(E) has combined with shifts in the demarcation of the public sector to almost radically alter

GO ON TO THE NEXT PAGE

16. Since the earliest times, women have been automatically denied vocational opportunity commensurate with men, and there are still far less women than men pursuing independent careers.

(A) men, and there are still far less women
(B) men's, and there are still far less of them
(C) that of men, and there are still far less women
(D) that of men, and there are still far fewer women
(E) those of men, and there are still far fewer women

17. Threatening their village, the bewildered and terrified peasants fled into the jungle while bombs and rockets burst nearby, gunships roared overhead, and wildly firing troops stormed across the paddies.

(A) Threatening their village, the bewildered and terrified peasants fled into the jungle while bombs and rockets burst nearby, gunships roared overhead, and wildly firing troops stormed across the paddies.
(B) While bombs and rockets burst nearby, gunships roared overhead, and wildly firing troops stormed across the paddies, at the threat to their village the bewildered and terrified peasants fled into the jungle.
(C) While bombs and rockets burst nearby, gunships roared overhead, and wildly firing troops stormed across the paddies, the bewildered and terrified peasants fled into the jungle at the threat to their village.
(D) At the threat to their village, the bewildered and terrified peasants fled into the jungle while bombs and rockets burst nearby, gunships roared overhead, and wildly firing troops stormed across the paddies.
(E) While bombs and rockets burst nearby, gunships roared overhead, and wildly firing troops stormed across the paddies, threatening their village, the bewildered and terrified peasants fled into the jungle.

18. The yellow jacket hornet is interesting to ecologists because clearly identifiable factors control its population and distribution, and not because of it being a serious pest to farmers and other country-dwellers.

(A) because of it being
(B) from the insect's being
(C) from its being
(D) because of its being
(E) because it is

19. Among the best qualified applicants for the position in the Department of Corrections are Rogers, Lopez, and Pulansky; the latter has even her doctorate in penology, as well as a master's degree in business administration.

(A) Pulansky; the latter has even her doctorate in penology, as well as
(B) Pulansky; Pulansky has even her doctorate in penology, plus having
(C) Pulansky, the last named even has her doctorate in penology, as well as
(D) Pulansky; the latter even has her doctorate in penology, in addition to
(E) Pulansky; the last named even has her doctorate in penology, in addition to

GO ON TO THE NEXT PAGE

20. The amazing multiplicity of Amerindian language families, established by a century of linguistic research, has not been satisfactorily explained by either linguistic or anthropological theory.

(A) families, established by a century of linguistic research,
(B) families, which linguists have established by a century of research,
(C) families, a phenomenon established by a century of linguistic research,
(D) families, being established by a century of linguistic research,
(E) families has been established by a century of linguistic research and

21. The government is sponsoring an income tax cut, but the congressional appropriations committee has not yet agreed upon a package of measures to offset the reduction in tax revenue.

(A) is sponsoring an income tax cut, but the congressional appropriations committee has not yet agreed upon
(B) is sponsoring an income tax cut, but the congressional appropriations committee have not yet agreed on
(C) are sponsoring an income tax cut, but the congressional appropriations committee has not yet agreed upon
(D) is sponsoring an income tax cut, but the congressional appropriations committee have not yet agreed
(E) is sponsoring an income tax cut, but the congressional appropriations committee have not yet agreed to

22. Her staff pleaded with the senator to delete much of the references to affirmative action in her keynote speech, a deletion which she did make, though loath to concede so much.

(A) to delete much of the references to affirmative action in her keynote speech, a deletion which she did make
(B) that she delete many of the references to affirmative action in her keynote speech, a deletion which was made by her
(C) to delete many of the references to affirmative action in her keynote speech, a deletion which she did make
(D) that she delete many of the references to affirmative action in her keynote speech, which she did delete
(E) to delete much of the references to affirmative action in her keynote speech, which she did

23. The governor ordered that the state police and the national guard jointly set up a cordon around the affected area, that passage through this cordon be authorized only by the state police commandant, and that only civil defense officials actually enter the area.

(A) passage through this cordon be authorized only by the state police commandant
(B) only the state police commandant authorizes passage through this cordon
(C) only the state police commandant authorize passage through this cordon
(D) passage through this cordon is authorized only by the state police commandant
(E) passage be authorized through this cordon only by the state police commandant

GO ON TO THE NEXT PAGE

24. Rather than to present in this introduction a detailed description of the collection, a description that will be given in the appendixes, it seems more useful to sketch here the highlights of this unique gallery.

(A) Rather than to present in this introduction a detailed description of the collection, a description that will be given in the appendixes, it seems more useful
(B) In this introduction it seems more useful, rather than presenting a detailed description of the collection and its contents, that will be given in the appendixes,
(C) In this introduction it seems more useful, rather than to present a detailed description of the collection and all its contents, which will be given in the appendixes,
(D) Rather than presenting in this introduction a detailed description of the collection, a description which will be given in the appendixes, it seems more useful
(E) Instead of presenting in this introduction a detailed description of the collection and its contents, a description that will be given in the appendixes, it seems more useful

25. It is especially significant that this material has been discovered in an aqueous environment, suggesting that intact neural tissue may be preserved in other than extremely arid conditions or permafrost, and greatly widening the sites to be probed for similarly ancient tissue.

(A) suggesting that intact neural tissue may be preserved in other than extremely arid conditions or permafrost, and greatly widening the
(B) because this discovery suggests that intact neural tissue may be preserved in other than extremely arid conditions or permafrost, and greatly increases the
(C) as this discovery suggests that intact neural tissue may be preserved in other than extremely arid conditions or permafrost, and greatly increases the number of
(D) suggesting that intact neural tissue may be preserved in other than extremely arid conditions or permafrost, and greatly widening the number of
(E) because it suggests that intact neural tissue may be preserved in other than extremely arid conditions or permafrost, and greatly increases the number of

End of Examination

STOP

YOU MAY CHECK YOUR WORK ON THIS SECTION ONLY UNTIL YOUR TIME IS UP.
DO NOT WORK ON ANY OTHER SECTION.

The

Answers and Explanations

to the FIRST EXAMINATION

begin on the next page.

The SECOND EXAMINATION begins on page 52.

Please refer back to the instructions on page 1

before starting work on this examination.

Answers to the First Examination

	Section I	Section II	Section III	Section IV	Section V	Section VI
1.	D	C	C	E	C	C
2.	A	E	A	C	E	A
3.	D	A	B	D	E	D
4.	C	C	C	A	D	B
5.	D	D	E	A	E	A
6.	E	B	D	D	C	A
7.	B	E	C	B	A	B
8.	C	C	E	E	E	D
9.	B	B	E	C	B	B
10.	C	D	B	A	C	E
11.	A	C	A	D	D	A
12.	B	C	E	E	A	B
13.	A	A	D	B	E	D
14.	E	D	B	D	D	E
15.	E	A	D	B	B	A
16.	C	E	A	A	A	D
17.	D	E	C	C	C	D
18.	A	A	B	B	D	E
19.	E	D	A	E	A	E
20.	B	B	E	D	E	C
21.	A		B	A		B
22.	E		D	C		C
23.	D		A	E		C
24.	B		D	B		A
25.	C		B	C		C

First Examination: Explanation of the Answers

Section I: Reading Comprehension.

1. The correct answer, D, reflects the main content and emphasis of the passage. The other choices relate to secondary and supporting ideas.

2. The correct answer, A, is most appropriate to the style and content of the passage. This content is basically nutritional information. The language of the passage is not technical enough to justify D or E, nor general enough to justify C.

3. The correct answer, D, is indicated by the words antagonist and administered in line 43. Glossitis and gastro-intestinal lesions are directly caused by "folacin deficiency" (line 41).

4. The correct answer, C, is supported by lines 5-7 and 10-11. In B, it is not human organs, but bacteria that synthesize folacin.

5. The correct answer, D, includes I, which is answered in lines 32-33, and III, which is answered extensively, e.g., in lines 37-38.

6. The correct answer, E, is justified by language such as "appears to" in line 10, "the difficulties ... in determining" in lines 12-13, and "may be important" in line 16.

7. The correct answer, B, may be inferred from lines 16-17: "experimental deficiency" especially suggests research in nutrition.

8. The correct answer, C, is supported by lines 9-11, the "inhibitor" being the natural substance mentioned. The other choices are non sequiturs.

9. The correct answer, B, can be inferred from the language (e.g., "pernicious," line 8) which Dexter applies to Williams' actions. B is supported also by the fact that Dexter is "the historian of Congregationalism" (line 7), the church against which Williams rebelled.

10. The correct answer, C, is most comprehensive. Central in the passage are the ramifications of Williams' heresies, and not his style of dissent, his Calvinism, or his critique of society. Lines 31-32 imply that he was not a civil libertarian.

11. The correct answer, A, is extensively implicit, e.g., in lines 21-22 and 32-33. B and C are much less forcefully implied.

12. The correct answer, B, is borne out, for example, by lines 32-41, in which Williams' shortcomings and virtues, from a modern viewpoint, are assessed and balanced.

13. The correct answer, A, may be inferred from lines 28-29. That D cannot be the answer may be inferred by juxtaposing line 5 and line 26; that E cannot be the answer may be inferred from lines 18-26.

14. The correct answer, E, may be inferred from lines 41-49. C is less strongly implied (e.g., in lines 23-26). A, B, and D are not implied.

15. The correct answer, E, may be inferred from the appropriate denotation of the word unregenerate as well as from the juxtaposition of lines 19-22 and lines 41-42.

16. The correct answer, C, may be inferred from the immediate context and from the conventions of the usage of quotation marks. These clues indicate that in line 25, as in line 27, the author is quoting seventeenth-century discourse.

17. The correct answer, D, may be inferred by putting together lines 22-26 and lines 45-49. It could be inferred that B, C, and E were considered objectionable by Williams' superiors, but these are less strongly implied to be threats.

18. The correct answer, A, best reflects the content and mode (exposition, not argument) of the passage. The introductory paragraph on classic economic theory is not central.

19. The correct answer, E, is borne out by lines 8-10 and 15-17. The other answer choices are borne out only partially, if at all, by the passage.

20. The correct answer, B, may be inferred by putting together lines 22-24 and lines 44-49. Lines 21-22, taken together with lines 36-39, imply that curing disease is considered a work of exploit.

21. The correct answer, A, may be inferred from the immediate context, which suggests the appropriate denotation of <u>assimilated to</u>.

22. The correct answer, E, includes II, which is explicitly stated in lines 12-15, and III, which is evident if one juxtaposes lines 21-22 and lines 29-31. I is ruled out by lines 22-24; IV is not mentioned in the passage.

23. The correct answer, D, expresses an idea neither stated nor implied in the passage. The other choices express ideas explicit in the passage.

24. The correct answer, B, is borne out in every sentence of the passage. The author expresses economic or anthropological concepts in a formal, polished style, without recourse to a technical vocabulary.

25. The correct answer, C, generalizes the closing idea that the phrase "brute matter" expresses a primitive conception. A and B are far-fetched inferences. Both D and E are misreadings.

<u>Section II: Problem Solving.</u>

1. The denominator of the fraction can be expresed as 4/12 + 3/12 which equals 7/12. The reciprocal of this value is the correct answer, 12/7, i.e., choice C.

2. Solution of the first equation gives $x = \frac{1}{4}$ and using this value in the second equation produces $\frac{1}{4}y = 4$ or $y = 8$, (choice E).

3. If A and B denote the amounts invested at $4\frac{1}{2}\%$ and 6%, respectively, then, A + B = 30,000 and 0.045A + 0.06B = 1,470. Solving the first equation for A, (A = 30,000 - B), and using this in the second equation yields: 0.045(30,000 - B) + 0.06B = 1,470, which simplifies to: 0.015B = 1,470 - 1,350. From this last equation, B can be found to be 120/0.015 = 8,000, i.e., choice A.

4. From the information given, a 2% decrease in CER produces a change of + 10 in the price index. It follows that an increase in the CER of 1% produces a change in the index of - 5. Combining this with the + 10 change due to the 1% increase in the AMR gives the net change, + 5, i.e., choice C.

5. If C and A represent the number of child and adult tickets bought respectively, then the answer, D, can be from the simultaneous solution of: $A - C = 50$ and $3A + C = 1,110$. Adding the two equations together gives $4A = 1160$ from which $A = 290$.

6. If DE is extended to intersect AB, two parallelograms are formed. The area of the smaller is $5(30) = 150$. The larger parallelogram has area $15(40) = 600$. Adding the two values together gives 750, answer B.

7. Diameter, d, of the circle equals the side of the larger square and is also the diagonal of the smaller square. The area of the larger square equals $2d^2$; the area of the smaller square = d^2. Therefore, the ratio of the areas is 2:1, (choice E).

8. Dividing 4,140° by 360° gives $11\frac{1}{2}$ rotations. The arrow comes to rest rotated 180° from its original direction, i.e., pointing at the black circle, choice C.

9. If X denotes the less expensive and Y the more expensive candy, then $X + Y = 60$ and $X(\$2/3) + Y(\$3/2) = 60(\$1)$. The second equation simplifies to $4X + 9Y = 360$; subtracting $4X + 4Y = 240$ from this, $5Y = 120$ or $Y = 24$, i.e., choice B.

10. Choice D is correct since $30 = (2)(3)(5)$, the product of three primes.

11. Repeated use of the Pythagorean theorem yields: $(AG)^2 = (AB)^2 + (BC)^2 + (CD)^2 + (DE)^2 + (EF)^3 + (FG)^2$. With the values given in the problem, $(AG)^2 = 6$ and this gives the correct choice, C.

12. The interest earned is one-half of $5\frac{1}{2}\%$ of 16,000 which is $\frac{1}{2}(0.055)(16000)$ or \$440. Adding this to the principal gives the correct choice, C.

13. From the first equation, $y = \frac{1}{2}x$. Using this in the second expression, gives $(\frac{1}{2}x^2 - x^2)/x^2 = -\frac{1}{2}x^2/x^2 = -\frac{1}{2}$ which is choice A.

14. Since there are 32 years difference between 1990 and 1958, the house value would have increased (2)(2)(2)(2) times. The 1990 value would be expected to be 16 times its 1956 value, i.e., \$128,000, choice D.

15. Each day, John can do one-ninth of the job. Together they get one-sixth of the job done each day. Paul's contribution must be $1/6 - 1/9$ or $1/18$ of the job each day. Consequently, Paul could do the job by himself in 18 days, choice A.

16. For the greatest value, the product, MN, must be negative (so that $-MN$ is positive). Therefore the greatest value will be either for $M = -5$ and $N = 11$ or for $M = 6$ and $N = -4$. These give either $M^2 - MN = 25 + 55 = 80$ and $M^2 - MN = 36 + 24 = 60$. The correct answer is E.

17. Choice E: if X is the original number of tables, then at the end of sale there remained 50% of two-thirds of 75% of 80% of X or $\frac{1}{2}(2/3)(3/4)(8/10)X$ which simplifies to $X/5$. Setting this equal to 18 and solving for X gives 90 as a result.

18. The sum of the angles of the five triangles is $(5)(180°) = 900°$. For each triangle, the angle whose vertex is located at the common point has a corresponding and equal angle opposite the triangle; therefore, at the common point, the sum of all angles inside the triangles equals the sum of those angles outside the triangles. Since the sum of these two sets of angles must equal 360°, it follows that the sum of those angles at the common point within triangles must be 180°. Consequently, the sum of the labeled angles must equal $900° - 180°$ or 720°. As there are 10 such angles, the average value must be $720°/10 = 72°$, choice A.

19. Choice D: path, DA, is the diagonal of a right triangle with sides 300+500 and 600, i.e., $800^2+600^2 = DA^2$; DA = 1000; added to 800 and 600, this gives 2400 meters.

20. Choice B is correct: to be divisible by 6, a number must be divisible by both 2 and 3, i.e., it must be an even number divisible by 3. Of the choices offered, only B and D are even numbers, and of these only choice B is divisible by 3.

Section III: Reading Comprehension.

1. The correct answer, C, best summarizes the content of the passage. B and D are too broad; A and E, too limited.

2. The correct answer, A, is borne out extensively in the author's argument (e.g., lines 24-33 and 44-46).

3. The correct answer, B, best interprets the relevant part of the passage (lines 1-5) and the use made of that part by the author.

4. The correct answer, C, is supported by lines 11-16 and by the inference from lines 5-11 that larceny was a "secondary offense." B seems attractive, but close reading reveals that the offender mentioned in lines 6-8 would be a layman claiming benefit of clergy, not an actual clergyman. Choice A may be ruled out by the distinction between hanging and prosecution.

5. The correct answer, E, may be inferred from the immediate context, in which the phrase in question is logically opposed to the subject of the following clause, i.e., reality.

6. The correct answer, D, includes II, which is answered in lines 25-29, and IV, which is answered in lines 24-25.

7. The correct answer, C, is a statement which runs counter to lines 39-42.

8. The correct answer, E, is borne out by lines 39-42 and 44-46.

9. Answer E best reflects the content and thrust of the passage.

10. The correct answer, B, is borne out by the general point of view of the passage (e.g., lines 23-25.)

11. The correct answer, A, is supported by lines 10-18, as well as by the implications of the concept of automatism in the passage. Choice B may be eliminated by distinguishing between delusion (not said to be found in post-hypnotic subjects) and hallucination (sometimes inducible by post-hypnotic suggestion, according to lines 15-17).

12. The correct answer, E, contains only III, which may be gathered from lines 18-23. Choice C seems attractive, but close reading reveals that "automatic" writing is not defined.

13. The correct answer, D, best interprets the phrase both in terms of the immediate context and in terms of the denotation of parasitic.

14. The correct answer, B, best reflects the tone of the passage, a tone illustrated, for example, in lines 32-34, which could be called confident, but not complacent.

15. The correct answer, D, may be inferred from lines 32-34. Choice A may seem attractive, but, in fact, the idea of repression is not implied by the author.

16. The correct answer, A, names something not found in the author's exposition. B, C, and E are found throughout the passage; D may be found, for example, in lines 6-7.

17. The correct answer, C, reflects the main pattern of exposition in the passage. Choice D is attractive, but it is not as comprehensive.

18. The correct answer, B, best describes the content and style of the passage, which continually returns to economic causes.

19. The correct answer, A, may be inferred by juxtaposing lines 15-17 and lines 26-35. The other answer choices are contradicted by the passage. Choice C is ruled out by the word plausible, an ascription contradicted by lines 11-14.

20. The correct answer, E, may be inferred from lines 2-4. The other answer choices are non sequiturs.

21. The correct answer, B, is not mentioned in the passage. The other answer choices are explicit in the passage.

22. The correct answer, D, may be inferred from the immediate context, as well as from the denotation of spurious.

23. The correct answer, A, is borne out by expressions such as "reputable wastefulness and futility" in line 15, "latest indigestible contrivance" in lines 31-32, and "intrinsic odiousness" in line 35. This tone cannot be described as either pedantic, self-righteous, humorless, or plaintive.

24. The best answer, D, is implicit throughout the passage (e.g., lines 10-14).

25. The correct answer, B, may be inferred from the main thrust of the passage, as well as from particular sentences such as lines 4-6.

Section IV: Data Sufficiency.

1. Using S, M, and L to represent the short, middle-size, and long pieces, then $L + 2M + S = 300$. From statement (1), it follows that either $S + M = 130$ and thus, $L + S = 170$. Using (2), gives $L + M + L = 170$ and $L - S = 40$, or $M = 65$ from which $L + S = 170$. Using (2), gives $L + 2M = 240$, which does not determine L. Equations (2) and (1) together, allow S, M, and L to be either 60, 65, 110 or 60, 70, 100. The correct answer is E.

2. The correct choice is C. If p is the original price per case, and q is the original number of cases sold, then $pq = \$2,000$. If the new price and quantity sold are P and Q respectively, then (1) gives $P = 0.9p$ and (2) gives $Q = 1.22q$. Using the two together, $PQ = (0.9)(1.22)pq = (0.9)(1.22)(\$2,000) = \$2,196$.

3. Since C is the center, $AC = BC$ and triangle ABC is an isosceles right triangle and arc AB is a quarter circle. From the value in (1), the formula for one-fourth the circumference of a circle gives a radius of 4. Therefore, AC and $BC = 4$ and the area is $\frac{1}{2}(4)(4) = 8$. From (2) alone, $BC = \frac{1}{2}(8) = 4$ and the area $= 8$ as before. The best answer is D.

4. From the statement of the problem, the height of the triangle = the x-coordinate of Q, i.e., $h = 6$. Statement (1) provides the length of the base, OP, as equal to 5 and the area can be determined as $\frac{1}{2}(6)(5) = 30$. Statement (2) provides no information on the length of OP; the correct choice is A.

5. The best choice is A: from statement (1), the total flow into the tank is 20 + 40 + 50 (= 110) gallons per minute. Since the slowest pipe provides 20 gal/min, the slowest pipe provides 20/110 of the entire volume or 18.2%. Statement (2), by itself, gives no information about the flow of the second pipe.

6. Choice D is correct. If y = x, then the line will be oriented at an angle of 45° to either the X or Y axes, therefore statement (1) is sufficient to answer the question. From the second statement (2), point B has coordinates which satisfies y = x. Since the origin, which also satisfies y = x, is on this line, statement (2), by itself, is also sufficient to answer the question.

7. Choice B: If L, W, and S equal the lengths of the length and width originally, and S is the side of the square plan, then from S = L - 3 and S = W + 1, statement (1), i.e., L = W + 4, can derived directly. From (2), the equation, (S + 3)(S - 1) = 96, reduces to $S^2 + 2S - 99 = 0$ which has roots, S = -11 and S = 9. Discarding the extraneous root, - 11, the area is 81 square meters.

8. Choice E: neither (1) nor (2) give sufficient information to determine the distance from B to line AC so the height (and the areas) cannot be determined.

9. Choice C: from (1), it follows two-thirds of the wheat and oat farmers must grow wheat, but the answer depends on the number of rye growers. From (2), it follows that there are 2,700 single-crop farmers who grow wheat or oats. Using both, 2/3 of 2,700 gives 1,800, a majority of the 3,000 farmers concerned.

10. Choice A: From (1), it follows that |x| is smaller than |y| and this is sufficient to answer the question. Statememt (2) gives no information about |y|.

11. The correct answer is D. From (1), 18 - 12 - 4 = 2 students must read more thar two newspapers. Therefore, these two readers are the only readers of three newspapers. From (2), there must be 30 - 19 - 9 = 2 readers of three newspapers.

12. Choice E: with no indication that angle BDC is a right triangle, there is insufficient information even with (1) and (2) to answer the question.

13. Statement (1) is insufficient to determine the sum of the numbers. From (2), the average can be calculated as 51/5 = 10.2; the best choice is B.

14. The correct choice is D. The problem infers that A = 2, B = 3, C = 5, D = 7, etc. Basically, the question becomes: is N divisible by 2? Since both statements (1) and (2) demonstrate that N is divisible by the even numbers 6 or 14, then either would answer the question.

15. Choice B. From the statement of the problem, $lw = 6x^2$, where lwh is the formula for the volume of a rectangular box. From (1) it follows that l = 3x and then w = 2x but no information is given about h. From (2) alone, it follows that the rectangular box must be 18 times the volume of the cube.

16. Choice A. From (1), it follows that x lies between 4.3 and 6.9 and since 5 is the only odd integer in that range, the question is answered. From (2), it follows that x is an odd number greater than 3.5 but this does not give a unique answer.

17. Choice C. From the problem, it can be determined that z = w + y. Using (1) alone, it follows that 2x = w + y but since w is unknown, the relative size of x and y cannot be determined. From (2) alone, adding y to both sides of the inequality gives z as being being greater than 3y or alternatively, y is less than one-third of z. Combining (1) and (2) yields y as less than one-third of (2x), i.e., y is less than two-thirds of x which answers the question.

18. The best choice is B. Using (1) alone, an answer depends on the value of n. From (2) alone, n must be an odd integer; consequently, for any value of x, the term, $(2 - x)^n$ must equal $-(x - 2)^n$. Therefore, the original expression will always equal 0.

19. Statement (1) is valid for the operators, +, ÷, and x. Statement (2) is valid for the mathematical operators, –, ÷, and x. Using both statements indicates that the operator can be x or ÷ and the correct choice is E.

20. Choice D. The sequence must be of the form: 7, 7N, $7N^2$, $7N^3$, $7N^4$, ... From (1), $7N^4 - 7N^3 = 4(7N^2 - 7N)$, from which, $N^2 = 4$. Since the fifth number in the sequence is $7N^4 = 7(4)^2 = 112$, statement (1) is sufficient. From (2): $(7N^2)(7N^3) = 14(7N^4)$ or $49N^5 = 98N^4$ from which N = 2 and $7N^4 = 112$.

21. From the statement of the problem, ABCD is a parallelogram and angle BAC equals angle ACD. From statement (1), AB = BC, from which ABC is an equilateral triangle with area $36\sqrt{3}$ which is half the area of ABCD. Statement (2) is a simple consequence of part of the original statement of the problem that AB ∥ DC. The best choice, therefore, is A.

22. The problem effectively asks if the number 12,3AB is divisible by both 3 and 4. Statement (1) guarantees that the sum of the digits of the original number would be a multiple of 3. Statement (2) guarantees that the number AB is a multiple of 4. Consequently, the two statements together answer the question, choice C.

23. Choice E. Statements (1) and (2) together are not sufficient as the 30 meters is not identified as being the longer or shorter side.

24. Choice B is correct. By expressing the term, x/y, as [1 + (x-y)/y] and the term, (x+3)/(y+3), as [1 + (x-y)/(y+3)], from (2), x-y is positive, and (x-y)/y is greater than (x-y)/(y+3) since the denominator of the former is smaller than the denominator of the latter. Without relative values of x and y, (1) is of no help.

25. Choice C is correct. From statement (1), K, L, and M shared 80 votes among them. From statement (2), K and L received 38 votes between them. Using (1) and (2) together gives 42 votes for M alone which answers the question.

Section V: Problem Solving.

1. The term within the brackets reduces to $\frac{3}{4}$; $(\frac{3}{4})^3$ is 27/64, choice C.

2. For the car with a loss, the $4,800 represented 3/4 of the cost; therefore, the cost of this car was (4/3)($4,800) = $6,400. For the car with a profit, $4,800 represented 125% of the cost; the cost was 4/5 of $4,800 = $3,840. Consequently, the combined cost of the two cars was $3,840 + $6,400 = $10,240 while the total amount received on the sale was 2 x $4,800 = $9,600. Thus, the dealer's net loss was $10,240 - $9,600 = $640. The correct choice is E.

3. If M represents the original number, then M = 100a + 10b + c, where a, b, and c represented the hundreds, tens, and units digits, respectively. The new number, N, formed by reversing the first and last digits, becomes N = 100c + 10b + a, and the difference, M – N, reduces to (M – N) = 99a – 99c. As this result is always a multiple of 99, the correct answer is E.

4. Pythagoras' theorem gives $AB^2 = 13^2 - 12^2$ and $BC^2 = 15^2 - 12^2$. From these equations, AB = 5 and BC = 9 which gives AC = 14; the correct choice is D.

5. From the problem statement, triangle ABC is isosceles and $x° = 180° - 5x°$. Solving this relationship gives the answer, $x = 30$, which is choice E.

6. The square root of $2^3 3^3 4^3 6^3 = 2(3)(4)(6)$ times the square root of $2(3)(4)(6)$, the latter term being the square root of $4(6)^2$. This becomes $2(3)(4)(6)[(2)(6)]$ which is $2^2(3)(4)6^2$, answer C.

7. Expansion of this expression gives $(/5)^2 + (/45)^2 - 2(/5)(/45)$. This simplifies to $5 + 45 - 2(15) = 50 - 30 = 20$. The correct answer is A.

8. The average speed for the two laps is the total distance divided by the total elapsed time. The average speed = $[10 + 10]/[(10/120)+(10/200)] = 20 \div [1/12 + 1/20] = 20[(20)(12)/(20 + 12)] = 20(20)(12)/32 = 150$ kph. The answer is choice E.

9. The numbers can be factored into $\frac{1}{2}(0.79 - 0.75)(0.79 + 0.75) = \frac{1}{2}(0.04)(1.54) = (0.02)(1.54) = 0.0308$. The best choice is B which is equivalent to 0.031.

10. If N and n represent the current and previous number, respectively, then the rule can be written: $N = 2n-1$. From this, the difference between the present and previous values, $N-n$, becomes: $N-n = n-1$. The problem infers that all numbers are different so $N-n$ cannot $= 0$, from which it follows, n cannot equal 1, choice C.

11. Using the normal conventions for coordinate axes, it follows that a, d, r and s must be negative. Of the choices, only D is not possible as bd is negative while r^2 is positive.

12. The problem reduces to $60^3/120^3$ which must be less than one, choice A.

13. If X is the amount of salt added, then the total amount of salt at the end, $X + 0.1(30)$, must be 25% of the final solution, $30 + X$. As an equation, this is $X + 3 = 7.5 + 0.25X$. Rearranging gives $0.75X = 4.5$, from which $X = 6$, choice E.

14. From the problem statement, $a° = x° + 2x° = 3x°$, then $b° = 5x°$, and $c° = 8x°$. Since $2x° + a° + b° + c°$ form a straight line, then $2x + 3x + 5x + 8x = 180$ and $18x = 180$ which gives $x = 10$. The largest angle, c, is 80°, choice D.

15. As its last digit is even, the original number is divisible by 2. Since the sum of its digits is 27, (a multiple of 9), the original number is also a multiple of 9; therefore, the original number can be divided by $2 \times 9 = 18$, choice B.

16. From the problem statement, ABC must be an isosceles triangle with angles A and B equal. Since C is 60°, A and B are 60° each and ABC is equilateral with sides of length 3. The shaded area and ABC have sides in the ratio of 1:3, therefore, the areas are in the ratio of 1:9. The areas of the unshaded region and area of ABC must be in the ratio of 8:9, which is equivalent to choice A.

17. From the problem, it follows that 90% of the cars are not black. For each color of car, the probability of randomly selecting an air-conditioned car with automatic transmission is $(0.8)(0.3) = 0.24 = 6/25$. Since 9/10 of these must be colors other than black, the final result is $(6/25)(9/10) = 27/125$, choice C.

18. In every 12 minutes, the pipe adds 6 kiloliters of water, and the drains empty 3 kiloliters and 2 kiloliters of water, respectively, with a net gain of 1 kiloliter every 12 minutes. Since 2 kiloliters of water are needed to fill the tank, it will take $2 \times 12 = 24$ minutes to fill the tank, answer D.

19. Angle d equals the unlabeled angle opposite it. Since this unlabeled angle added to e, a, b, and c form a straight line, it follows that $a + b + c + d + e = 180$. In the diagram, $e = 47$, then $a + b + c + d = 180 - 47 = 133$, i.e., choice A.

20. To find the area, the length of the remaining side, x, must be determined from the Pythagorean theorem. This gives $x^2 = (6\frac{1}{2})^2 - 6^2$ or $x^2 = 42.25 - 36 = 6.25$ and from this, x = 2.5. The area is 2.5 x 6 = 15, choice E.

Section VI: Sentence Correction.

1. In the correct answer, C, both verbs agree with the plural subject, types. Choices A, D, and E err in agreement; choices E and B introduce misrelated participial phrases.

2. The best answer, A, is the clearest and most concise statement. Choices B and E are wordy, while authoress in E might be objected to as a usage patronizing to women. The use of the passive voice in C is awkward and confusing. In D the pronoun she has no antecedent.

3. The correct choice, D, uses the past perfect tense and the infinitive with the verb intend. All the other choices fail to use the infinitive to intend, while choices B and E fail to follow tense sequence.

4. The correct choice, B, has a singular verb because the antecedent of who is member, not board. Moreover, Martinez' must be in the possessive case because it is the subject of the gerund getting. Choice D, the only other choice to get these points correct, introduces the unidiomatic is opposing to.

5. The best answer, A, expresses the three measurements in parallel form with acceptable phrasing. Choices B and C not only lack parallelism but also introduce the redundant in shape. In D, as to shape is both redundant and substandard. The expressions of measurement in choice E are nonstandard and lack apostrophes to indicate possessive form.

6. In the correct answer, A, the adjective, largest, is used in the superlative degree to indicate one among many. Moreover, the verb must be forage to agree with the plural antecedent of that, namely, genera. In E, the participle foraging is inferior to that forage as an expression of a trait.

7. The correct choice, B, subordinates and contrasts the idea in the first clause to that in the second. Choices A and E seem awkward and illogical because they fail to contrast the two clauses. Choices C and D correctly contrast the two clauses, but they fail to use the past perfect tense, had ... emigrated, the tense called for by the context.

8. The correct choice, D, compares the weight of a bear to that of two lions. Choice E illogically compares weight and lions. Choices A and B contain awkward double genitives; those in A is not parallel with weight; and the last word of B is redundant. In C, the last word is also redundant, and the form of the plural possessive is incorrect.

9. The best answer, B, is precise in the word order of not only ... but also. In D, not only is illogically placed before carries. In A and E, the verb assures is incorrectly used intransitively. Moreover, choices A, C, and E awkwardly introduce a second clause following not only; and the pronoun it and the phrase the student in these choices are vague.

10. The best choice is E. In choices A and D, the use of the idiom due to to mean because of is considered colloquial. Choice B avoids this mistake but is otherwise garbled. In choice C, the idiom consequent on is stilted and the parenthetical phrase in which it appears is an unnecessary complication of the sentence.

11. The correct answer, A, is parallel in grammatical form to the first two items in the series, namely, reception and issuance. Choice B is wordy and choices C, D, and E introduce a gerund.

12. The correct answer, B, follows the rule that the indefinite antecedent each is construed as singular. In addition, expressions of general truth, especially in American English, are put in the present tense.

13. The best answer, D, relates the introductory participle phrase to its subject, managers, and D uses the present perfect form have shown to express an action begun in the past and continuing into the present. Choices A and B are correct only in respect to tense; E is correct in sentence structure but is not correct in tense.

14. The correct choice, E, introduces a main clause parallel to the first main clause. Choices A, B, and D awkwardly shift to the passive voice, resulting in vagueness and redundancy. Choice C introduces a misrelated participial phrase.

15. The correct choice, A, makes the verb has agree with its subject, deregulation; and choice A places the phrase almost radically in a position where the meaning of the phrase is clear. Choices B and E awkwardly split the infinitive to alter.

16. The correct answer, D, compares opportunity with that of men, and choice D appropriately qualifies the count noun women. Choice A illogically compares opportunity and men. Choice E imprecisely compares opportunity (singular) with those of men. Moreover, choices A, B, and C apply the quantitative adjective less to the count noun women.

17. In the correct choice, D, the word order is most effective. In choices A and E the participial phrase threatening their village is dangling. In B and C, the word order is awkward and anticlimactic.

18. In the correct answer, E, the conjunctive expression and not is followed by a clause which balances the previous clause beginning with because. The other answer choices introduce an awkward gerund phrase, and choice A fails to put the subject of that phrase, it, in the possessive case.

19. The correct choice, E, avoids the misuse of latter, a word which properly refers to the last mentioned of two items. Choice B introduces the awkward, misrelated phrase plus having. Choice C incorrectly links the main clauses with a comma (instead of a semicolon). Choices A and B misplace the adverb even.

20. Choice C is best because it is clearest. Choice A does not make clear what has been established, multiplicity or families. Choices B and D aggravate this problem: choice B uses the vague which and choice D uses the redundant being. Choice E avoids this ambiguity, but its compound predicate is too long and it co-ordinates two ideas which are not equal in importance.

21. In American English, government is construed as singular. In the correct choice, B, the plural verb have is used correctly with the collective noun committee. In C, has is singular. In D, the agreement is correct, but agreed lacks a preposition to complete its meaning. In E, agreed to not only changes the meaning of the statement, but also conflicts with the plural meaning of committee.

22. The best answer is C. In A and E, the quantitative noun much incorrectly refers to the count noun, references. In D and E, which is ambiguous. Choice B awkwardly shifts to the passive voice in the last four words, and B and D introduce misrelated noun clauses.

23. In the correct choice, C, parallel structure is observed in the active voice; and the subjunctive form, authorize, follows the expression of command. This use of the subjunctive mood is more common in American English than in British English. (Note that in A the subjunctive form is correct, though the passive voice of A is not parallel.) In choice E, apart from errors in parallelism and subjunctive form, the word order, especially the position of only, is confusing.

24. The correct answer, A, exhibits parallel structure and clear word order. Choices B, D, and E violate parallel structure by matching a gerund, presenting, with the following infinitive, to sketch. Choice E also contains the redundancy, and its contents. Choice C has the redundancy and all its contents, a confusing word order, and an ambiguous which. Choice B combines a faulty word order with an incorrect use of the relative pronoun that in a nonrestrictive clause. Choice B also contains the redundancy and its contents.

25. In the correct answer, C, the cause-and-effect relationship of the parts of the sentence is sustained in the subordinate clause beginning with as. Choices A and D introduce a participial phrase beginning with suggesting which is not clearly related, either grammatically or logically, to the rest of the sentence. Also, choice A omits number of; and widening in A and D makes no sense. In choices B and E, the construction is correct, but B omits number of. In E, it is ambiguous; here it could refer either to the material or to the fact that the material has been discovered.

The

SECOND EXAMINATION

begins on the page 52.

Please refer back to the instructions on page 1

before starting work on this examination.

Section I

Time - 30 minutes

25 Questions

Directions: Each passage in this group is followed by questions on content. After reading a passage, choose the best answer to each question and blacken the corresponding space on the answer sheet. Answer all questions following a passage on the basis of what is stated or implied in that passage.

In modern behavioral genetics, genotype is considered to operate with environmental factors to produce phenotype or observed behavior characteristics. Combined with newer quantitative genetics, this approach offers vastly improved understanding of individual differences in behavior.
(5) Throughout the organism's development and lifespan, genetic influence is being expressed. The genetic material (deoxyribonucleic acid or DNA) sends its messages in a form of ribonucleic acid (RNA) into the cytoplasm of cells. Copies of each form of RNA determine specificity of enzymes. These enzymes in turn are responsible for physiological functioning.
(10) Characteristics of the central nervous system, sensory systems, and other systems such as the effectors and the endocrines are influenced by nutritional and other environmental biochemical factors. Where the resulting interaction with the environment is favorable, the organism survives and reproduces. We cannot over-emphasize the contributions of our
(15) biological heritage toward the establishment of these genetic potentials for adaptation. While most of the science of genetics has developed from the study of infrahuman forms, we will concentrate on what can be applied to human biology and behavior.
A fundamental principle pervading all recent data on environmental
(20) effects is that of variations in optimum environments. The best environment for a given individual may be importantly different from that for another individual because of innate endowments. Illustrations of biochemical differences are numerous. The so-called normal population varies in its response to specific reward systems. Food and temperature preferences,
(25) dietary requirements, and tolerance for toxins all vary rather widely. Some individuals are unable to metabolize certain essential amino acids. In individuals deficient in the liver enzyme, phenylalanine hydroxylase, the essential amino acid, phenylalanine, is not converted into tyrosine. This failure harms the developing nervous system. The IQ of children suffering
(30) from this genetic malady is typically below 50. Altering the diet is partially successful in reducing the effects of this biochemical deficiency. Less dramatic and not always as clear are some 30 other conditions in which urine testing may uncover metabolic dysfunction. Further research is urgently needed in order to advance our knowledge and pediatric control over
(35) these conditions.
Certain of our measurable behavioral traits respond strongly to environmental variables, while others respond only when there are appropriate genetic supports. In recent studies of intellectual functions, the degree of genetic determination appears to be quite high or quite low
(40) depending upon the function. Vandenberg reports a strong genetic component in number and fluency traits, space and verbal conceptualization, and personality traits like emotionality, activity level, and introversion. However, reasoning and memory appear to have little or no genetic component.

GO ON TO THE NEXT PAGE

1. The author's main purpose in this passage is to

(A) argue that environmental factors are less important than genetic factors in determining mental traits
(B) analyze the basis of modern behavioral genetics
(C) outline the factors influencing our measurable behavioral traits
(D) maintain that genetic and environmental factors are equally balanced in determining the organism's development
(E) indicate that the organism's development consistently reflects the interaction of genetic and environmental factors

2. Which of the following statements about the older genetic approaches to individual differences in behavior CANNOT be inferred from the first paragraph of the passage?

(A) the older approaches fell far short of the modern approach
(B) the older approaches confused genotype and phenotype
(C) the older approaches failed to study the interaction of genetic and environmental influences
(D) the older approaches did not make use of quantitative genetics
(E) the older approaches have been superseded

3. In the second paragraph of the passage, which sentence has least relation to the main topic of that paragraph?

(A) the sentence beginning, "Throughout the organism's development ... "
(B) the sentence beginning, "The genetic material ... "
(C) the sentence beginning, "These enzymes ... "
(D) the sentence beginning, "Where the ... "
(E) the sentence beginning, "While most ... "

4. The passage contains information to answer which of the following questions?

I. How does genotype influence the adult person's physiology?
II. What effect does deficiency in phenylalanine hydroxylase have upon the metabolic capability of the developing child?
III. Does available evidence show that a good memory is hereditary?

(A) I, II, and III
(B) I and II only
(C) I and III only
(D) II and III only
(E) III only

5. In line 17, the phrase "infrahuman forms" most exactly refers to

(A) abnormal or pathological cases
(B) cells and tissues removed from animals
(C) plants and animals
(D) extrapolations from intensive studies of individuals
(E) anthropoid apes

GO ON TO THE NEXT PAGE

6. According to the passage, the optimum environment of one person may differ considerably from that of another person, because

(A) the persons may differ in their genetic constitutions
(B) the population varies in its response to food and temperature requirements
(C) the persons may differ in their phenotypes
(D) the persons may exhibit differing metabolic dysfunctions or other physiological conditions
(E) genotypes cannot respond to environmental variables

7. All of the following may be inferred from the passage EXCEPT that

(A) tyrosine is an enzyme affecting the development of IQ
(B) the ability to express ideas in words seems to be influenced by heredity
(C) nutritional factors may play a role in the development of nervous disorders
(D) both personality and intelligence are influenced by genetic factors
(E) there is a genetic component in the varying abilities of people to tolerate poisons

8. It may be inferred from the last paragraph of the passage that the influence of hereditary factors upon mental abilities

(A) is directly related to environmental variables
(B) can be determined only if the ability in question is measurable
(C) varies according to the respective personality traits
(D) varies considerably from one ability to another
(E) depends upon whether an ability is verbal or quantitative

While some laymen and all social scientists speak of role, many persons find they have the same problem with this term that St. Augustine faced when dealing with the concept of time: he knew what it was until asked to define it. I find that a statistical-probability approach helps fix the concept of (5) role for persons inexperienced in the social sciences. Human behavior is not random; that is, consistencies exist in human behavior. These consistencies may characterize the behavior of an individual over many activities as parent, spouse, or worker. When we look at the consistencies of a pervasive behavior we are considering a psychological variable, and we (10) are not concerned with the concept of role as such. Johnny may be bright or dull, paranoid or not paranoid, confident or not confident across many or all of his different behaviors.

However, there are consistencies in human behavior which characterize groups of persons in a society, regardless of their personal characteristics. (15) There are ways mothers, fathers, spouses, or members of an ethnic group behave and which do not, per se, have anything to do with personal characteristics. Therefore, if we are considering the consistencies of a person's behavior across many activities (i.e., roles), we are dealing with a psychological variable. But if we are considering the consistencies of a (20) type of behavior (e.g., mothering) across many persons, we are dealing with a sociological variable. It is to these consistencies within a type of behavior across many persons that sociologists give the name of role.

GO ON TO THE NEXT PAGE

We can now move to a more common definition of role as one part of the reciprocal set of human relationships characterized by a reciprocal set of
(25) rights and duties, as in the "rules" defining the relationship between mother and child, teacher and student, employer and employee. These rules are mainly defined before the child is born, before the student enters the classroom, or the employee the factory.

Therefore, if we wish to locate roles in order to measure them, we must
(30) look to the expectations people have about behavior. These expectations may exist at the level of belief regarding one's rights and duties in a human relationship (at one end of the continuum), or these expectations may exist at the level of patterned reflexes, as in the infant's interaction with his mother. The point is that roles lie suspended in the expectations or
(35) beliefs that people have about some given human interaction.

It is this fact that makes the concept of role so abstract and seemingly difficult to grasp. For while calories, vitamins, neurons, and synapses are easily reified and even such psychological abstractions as personality, intelligence, or need for achievement are often treated as if they had some
(40) sort of concrete, individual existence, it is impossible to think of role as a purely individual phenomenon.

9. In this passage the author's main purpose is to

(A) define a methodology
(B) delineate a concept
(C) propose a hypothesis
(D) refute a theory
(E) contrast two approaches

10. In the first paragraph, the reference to St. Augustine's problem with the concept of time is most probably intended to

(A) warn the reader of the intractable difficulties of conceptualization to be discussed
(B) give some indication of the historical background of the following discussion
(C) prepare the reader to grasp a similar problem in defining a familiar but elusive concept
(D) intimate that abstractions such as time or role have been adequately defined only by modern social scientists
(E) suggest that definitions of philosophical concepts have always contained ambiguities

11. The passage contains information to answer which of the following questions?

I. How does a psychological variable differ from a sociological variable?
II. What are some of the "rules" implicit in reciprocal human relationships?
III. Which patterned reflexes inhibit role?

(A) I, II, and III
(B) I and II only
(C) I and III only
(D) I only
(E) II and III only

GO ON TO THE NEXT PAGE

12. In the context of the passage, which of the following could best be substituted for the word reified (line 38)?

(A) pictured as material objects
(B) defined as biological entities
(C) described in scientific terms
(D) conceived as abstractions
(E) considered as symbolic units

13. It can be inferred from the passage that all of the following are examples of sociological role behavior EXCEPT

(A) a Victorian father instructing his children to address him as "Sir"
(B) a freshman obeying a command to stand on his head during a fraternity initiation
(C) a salesman offering a prospective customer an expensive cigar
(D) a wife ironing her husband's shirts
(E) a woman exhibiting extreme nervousness at a cocktail party

14. The author's attitude towards laymen or non-specialists could best be described as

(A) superior but patronizing
(B) impatient and a little contemptuous
(C) indifferent or dismissive
(D) frank and understanding
(E) humorous but detached

15. It may be inferred from the passage that

(A) sociological role is a difficult concept to grasp because it is not quantifiable or measurable
(B) role behavior depends upon the individual traits of each member of a given group or reciprocal relationship
(C) psychological abnormalities are irrelevant in analyses of role behavior
(D) role behavior is less predictable than is an individual's behavior across many activities
(E) ethical principles have little to do with role behavior

16. In the context of the passage, the point that "roles lie suspended in the expectations or beliefs that people have about some given human interaction" (lines 34-35) may best be taken to mean that

(A) role behavior is determined by collective attitudes and patterns of interaction
(B) a person's behavior in any given situation is based on what is expected by others
(C) sociological variables determine social behavior
(D) social activity may be aborted by the pressure of the peer group
(E) a person's behavior in any given interaction with other persons is based upon antecedent conditions

GO ON TO THE NEXT PAGE

Ignatius Donnelly's novel Caesar's Column (1891) projects a dystopian vision of American society in 1988. At first glance, New York is a smokeless, noiseless, glass-roofed dream city. But we soon discover that the city, like the nation at large, is engaged in a deadly social conflict
(5) between a ruling oligarchy, which maintains a dirigible fleet armed with gas bombs, and a rebellious urban proletariat joined by a persecuted peasantry. The story climaxes in the total breakdown of the social order after the looting and burning of the city by revolutionaries called the Brotherhood of Destruction rages beyond the oligarchy's control. So many corpses litter
(10) the streets that an immense pyramid of them is cemented over, as both sanitary precaution and memorial. Finally the entire city is put to the torch, destroying everyone except a small band of socialists who escape to Africa.

The novel's apocalyptic fury relates directly to the political hysteria
(15) of the 1880's — to the fears of anarchy, for example, that swept the nation after the Haymarket riot in Chicago in 1886, and to the bloody Homestead and Pullman strikes a few years later. Caesar's Column is also a striking prophecy of the events of the summer of 1967 in Newark and Detroit. But even while noting these resemblances between literature and life, we must
(20) confront the important difference, which is that the novel is much more extreme than the reality. Donnelly was no mere seismograph, passively recording social shocks, or even forecasting them; rather, he was a man driven to write by the experience of political loss, and the darkness of his apocalyptic vision tells us more about his state of mind than about America,
(25) past or present.

A Minnesotan political reformer staggered by the corruption of his state's legislature, Donnelly was also a Populist, worried by both the deteriorating economic position of the Midwestern farmer and the indications that America was becoming dominated by its big cities. He saw that the
(30) current demographic trends would reduce the importance of the farm vote and spread the spirit of corruption. In equating urbanism and corruption, and in envisioning damnation and destruction as the ultimate penalty of city life, Donnelly proved himself, in Richard Hofstadter's judgment, both sadist and nihilist. Caesar's Column is a "childish book," Hofstadter has written,
(35) "but in the mid-twentieth century it seems anything but laughable; it affords a frightening glance into the potential of frustrated popular revolt." The novel is thus for Hofstadter a key to the provincial spirit of Midwestern America, a spirit ruled by suspicion of Easterners and intellectuals, hatred of Jews, and fantasies of Babylonian destruction. The
(40) novel's violence may never have been matched by the social data of American history, but Hofstadter would contend that the American hick's sado-nihilism is inescapable in our civilization's emotional actuality, and that Donnelly's novel expresses a profoundly dangerous phenomenon.

17. In this passage the analysis of Caesar's Column is mainly concerned with

(A) contrast of appearance and reality
(B) social and cultural implications
(C) historical background
(D) autobiographical elements
(E) style, imagery, and motif

GO ON TO THE NEXT PAGE

18. In the context of the passage, the phrase "dystopian vision" (lines 1-2) refers most directly to

(A) socioeconomic analysis
(B) contrast of past and present
(C) surreal portrayal of anarchy
(D) pessimistic prediction
(E) cinematic technique

19. It may be inferred from the passage that Caesar's Column is characterized by which of the following?

I. a deceptively utopian view of New York City
II. references to the Haymarket riot
III. a turgid style and apocalyptic vision
IV. an unflattering delineation of "the American hick"

(A) I, II, III, and IV
(B) II and IV only
(C) I and III only
(D) I and IV only
(E) I only

20. It can be inferred that the author of the passage would find most rewarding which of the following research projects?

(A) a correlation of statistics on political violence and novel-reading in late nineteenth-century America
(B) a stylistic analysis of the portrayal of violence and sadism in all of Donnelly's novels
(C) an analysis of Cold War attitudes as revealed in American comic strips of the 1940s and '50s
(D) a detailed comparison of Caesar's Column and important nineteenth-century European political novels
(E) a survey of the socioeconomic implications of all American novels published during the 1890s

21. It can be inferred from the passage that Hofstadter would agree with all of the following observations EXCEPT that

(A) Donnelly derived a morbid pleasure from describing the holocaust of New York City
(B) Caesar's Column would be laughable except that its author denounces the more threatening aspects of the spirit of popular revolt
(C) Donnelly believed that metropolises were inherently evil
(D) American culture harbors destructive and xenophobic tendencies
(E) Caesar's Column reveals more than its author intended

22. In the light of the passage, the author might most consistently apply which of the following metaphoric ascriptions to Donnelly?

(A) a Jeremiah
(B) a social barometer
(C) a bellwether
(D) a Jonah
(E) a scapegoat

GO ON TO THE NEXT PAGE

23. It can be inferred from the passage that the author and Hofstadter are in basic agreement on all of the following EXCEPT

(A) the monitory significance of Caesar's Column
(B) what Caesar's Column reveals about American civilization
(C) the value of pursuing cultural analyses of literary texts
(D) the character of Donnelly
(E) the historical data of Donnelly's biography

24. In the passage the word apocalyptic is applied to Caesar's Column, because the novel

(A) is a vehicle of a radicalism that is both social and cultural
(B) exhibits a diseased imagination in its distortion of reality
(C) expresses a cryptic revelation symbolically
(D) is obsessed with themes and imagery of violence and cruelty
(E) climaxes in a retributive holocaust

25. It may be inferred from the passage that Donnelly himself was probably most sympathetic to which of the following?

(A) nihilism
(B) socialism
(C) anarchy
(D) anti-Semitism
(E) oligarchy

STOP

YOU MAY CHECK YOUR WORK ON THIS SECTION ONLY UNTIL YOUR TIME IS UP.
DO NOT WORK ON ANY OTHER SECTION.

SECTION II

Time - 30 minutes

20 Questions

Directions: In this section solve each problem, using any available space on the page for scratchwork. Then indicate the best answer of the answer choices given.

Numbers: All numbers used are real numbers.

Figures: Figures that accompany problems in this text are intended to provide information useful in solving the problem. They are drawn as accurately as possible EXCEPT when it is stated in a specific problem that its figure is not drawn to scale. All figures lie in a plane unless otherwise indicated.

1. A farmer's orchard was planted with 40 trees in a rectangular pattern, 10 trees to a row. Due to very cold weather, the last tree in each row dies and later the farmer replants some of the remaining trees in a pattern with equal rows and columns. What was the smallest number of trees that must be replanted?

   (A) 4 (B) 8 (C) 12 (D) 18 (E) 36

2. The expression $\frac{w\,x^3y^5z^7}{w^7x^5y^3z} =$

   (A) $\frac{y^2z^7}{x^7w^2}$ (B) $\frac{y^2z^6}{w^6x^2}$ (C) $(wxyz)^{16}$

   (D) $\frac{yz^8}{wx}$ (E) $\frac{z^3y^2}{wx}$

3. The fraction $\frac{(0.375)(2.51)(3.99)}{3(0.49)(0.53)}$ is approximately equal to

   (A) 5 (B) 4 (C) $\frac{9}{4}$ (D) $\frac{4}{3}$ (E) $\frac{1}{3}$

4. If a, b, and c are consecutive positive integers greater than 20, what is the largest integer, x, such that $\frac{abc}{x}$ is an integer?

   (A) 10 (B) 8 (C) 6 (D) 4 (E) 2

5. If $\frac{2}{3} \cdot \frac{4}{5} \cdot \frac{6}{7} \cdot \frac{3}{8} \cdot \frac{5}{6} \cdot k = 1$

   then k =

   (A) 14 (B) 19 (C) 9 (D) 7 (E) 1

GO ON TO THE NEXT PAGE

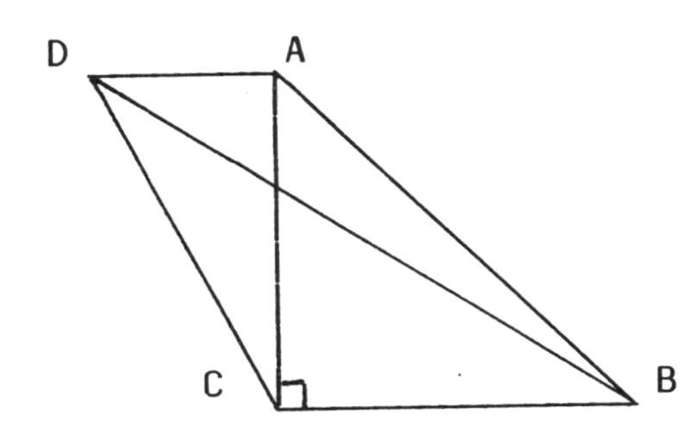

6. Triangle ABC has an area of 72 square meters and DA || CB. If angle ABC is 45° and AD equals 5 meters, how long, in meters, is CD?

(A) 12 (B) 13 (C) 15 (D) 17 (E) 23

7. If a mathematical operator, * , is defined by the relationships,

$$x * y = \frac{(x - y)^2}{(x + y)^2}, \quad (x + y) \neq 0,$$

which of the following must be true?

I: $0 * y = 1$

II: $x * y = y * x$

III: $x * \frac{1}{y} = \frac{1}{x} * y$

(A) I (B) II (C) I and II
(D) I and III (E) I, II, and III

8. If $-4 < a < 3$ and $7 > x > 3$, what is the range of all possible values of a(ax)?

(A) $-48 < a(ax) < 63$
(B) $0 \leqslant a(ax) < 63$
(C) $0 \leqslant a(ax) < 112$
(D) $27 \leqslant a(ax) < 63$
(E) $27 \leqslant a(ax) < 112$

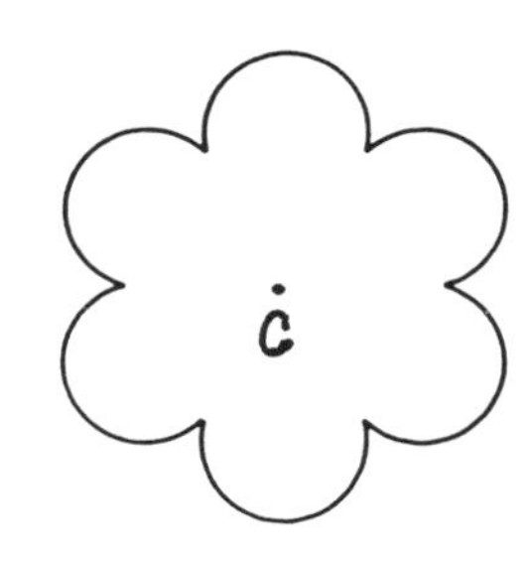

9. The figure above was formed by joining the ends of 6 equal semi-circles. If R is the distance from the center, C, to the intersections of the semi-circles, what is the total length of the perimeter of the figure?

(A) πR (B) $2\pi R$ (C) $3\pi R$
(D) $4\pi R$ (E) $6\pi R$

10. A computer salesman sells an average of 15 computer systems a month at $4,200 per system. He earns a basic salary of $22,000 per year plus a commission of $7\frac{1}{2}$% on monthly sales made over a level of $25,000 per month. What is his expected annual income?

(A) $78,700
(B) $75,200
(C) $66,700
(D) $56,200
(E) $34,200

GO ON TO THE NEXT PAGE

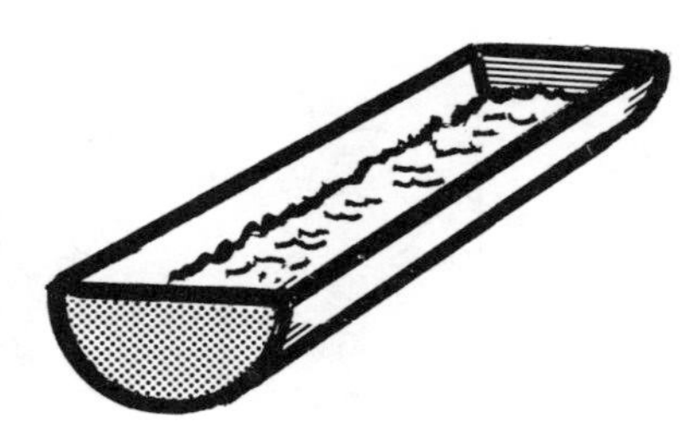

11. A water tank, made from an enclosed cylinder cut in half lengthwise, is filled to two-thirds of its capacity. The water is then allowed to drain into a cylindrical barrel standing on end. If the diameter of the barrel is twice the diameter of the water tank, and the original water tank was 480 centimeters long, then the depth of the water in the barrel, in centimeters, is

    (A) 40 (B) 80 (C) 120
    (D) 160 (E) 240

12. The value of y for which $y^2 + 6 = 5y$ and $7y - y^2 = 12$ is:

    (A) -1 (B) 0 (C) 1 (D) 2 (E) 3

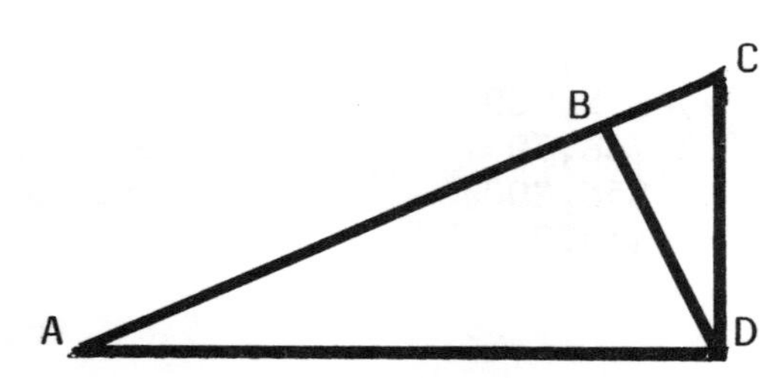

13. In right triangle ACD, AD = 12, CD = 5, and BD is perpendicular to AC. The length, BD, equals

    (A) $\frac{12}{5}$ (B) $\frac{144}{25}$ (C) 4
    (D) $\frac{60}{13}$ (E) 6

14. If the integer, N, is divided by 8, the remainder is 4. Which of the following is a multiple of 6 ?

    (A) $N + 2$
    (B) $6N + 9,876,543$
    (C) $3N + 9$
    (D) $\frac{1}{2}N - 1$
    (E) $\frac{3}{4}N + 3$

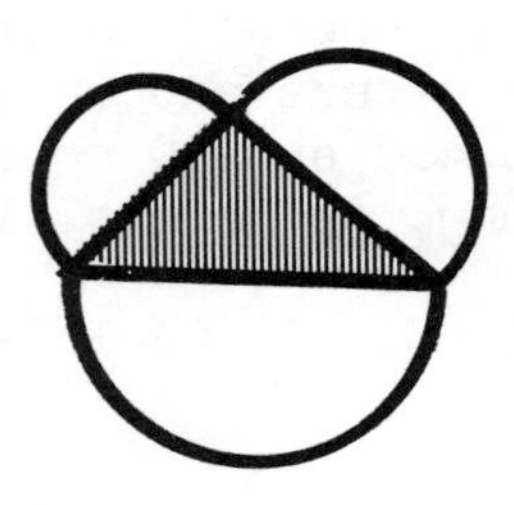

15. In the figure above, the curved border is made up of semi-circles constructed on the three sides of a triangle having lengths, a, b, and c. What is the ratio of the perimeter of the curved border to the perimeter of the triangle?

    (A) $\frac{\pi}{2}$ (B) π (C) $\frac{3\pi}{2}$ (D) 2π

    (E) cannot be determined from the information given

16. The expression

    $\frac{1}{4}(x^2 + y^2) - \frac{1}{2}(x + y)^2 + \frac{1}{2}xy =$

    (A) xy (B) 0 (C) $\frac{1}{4}(x^2 - y^2)$

    (D) $\frac{-(x + y)^2}{4}$

    (E) $\frac{(4xy - x^2 - y^2)}{4}$

GO ON TO THE NEXT PAGE

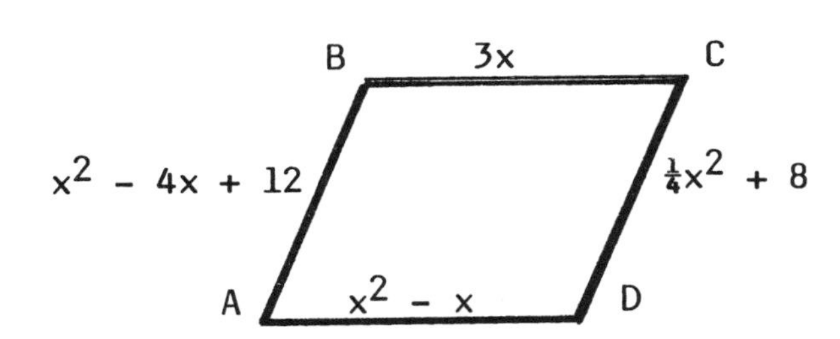

17. In the parallelogram ABCD with sides of length shown in the figure above, AB = BC. What is the length of side AB?

(A) 12 (B) 10 (C) 8 (D) 6 (E) 4

18. The average (arithmetic mean) of the three numbers, 64, 65, 66, is how many times larger than the average (arithmetic mean) of the five numbers, 11, 12, 13, 14, 15 ?

(A) $\frac{7}{5}$ (B) $\frac{5}{3}$ (C) 3 D) $\frac{22}{5}$ (E) 5

19. A circle is divided into twelve equal pie-shaped pieces and every other piece is shaded. If the circle has a diameter of 12, what is the total area of the shaded pieces?

(A) 36π (B) 18π (C) 12π (D) 6π (E) 3π

20. A chemist adds pure alcohol to a mixture containing 10% alcohol to make a mixture that contains 25% alcohol. The increase in volume represents what percentage change in the original mixture?

(A) 15% (B) 20% (C) 25% (D) 30% (E) 35%

STOP

YOU MAY CHECK YOUR WORK ON THIS SECTION ONLY UNTIL YOUR TIME IS UP.
DO NOT WORK ON ANY OTHER SECTION.

Section III

Time - 30 minutes

20 Questions

Directions: For each question in this section, select the best of the answer choices given.

1. In common with other scientists, the linguists who study language and culture avoid value judgements. This attitude has led to the rather uncomfortable situation in which the word "culture" in the vocabulary of these scientists refers to the social structure of the simplest communities, whereas for most other people it applies to the sophisticated products of advanced societies.

   Which of the following statements could be inferred from the above?

   (A) Value judgements apply only to highly civilized communities.
   (B) Linguists prefer to study primitive communities.
   (C) Linguists, in common with other scientists, present the data they collect without coming to any conclusions about them.
   (D) Value judgements obscure scientific findings.
   (E) A linguist would have nothing to say about the Mona Lisa.

2. Megalithic building went on for perhaps several thousand years, and throughout this period, the ideas governing the erection of stones must not have been static. During periods of political stability, an increase in knowledge by natural development or by diffusion from elsewhere would probably be reflected in the stones. The cruder circles were most likely earlier - we must be prepared to find indications of growth at some sites where perhaps one scheme was being replaced by another. Such development can be expected in the geometry and in the knowledge of astronomy.

   With which of the following statements would the author agree?

   (A) The making of stone circles led to the development of astronomy.
   (B) It is likely that the purpose of megaliths was seen differently by the successive peoples who reworked the sites.
   (C) We can deduce evidence of political activity from the megaliths.
   (D) Stone circles can provide a prehistoric record of peace and war covering thousands of years.
   (E) The more civilized people have become, the larger they make their megaliths.

3. The boy says to his father, "I don't want to eat those peas, because they will give me a stomach ache. I got a stomach ache every time I ate peas last week."

   The argument above is most nearly like which of the following?

   (A) The reduction in fossil fuel reserves predicted by the study shows an urgent need for the development of alternative energy sources.
   (B) The painting cannot be a Rembrandt because the pigments used are found only in portraits painted subsequent to Rembrandt's death.
   (C) The skin rash is caused by the new brand of soap used, since every person in the sample using the soap developed a skin rash later on.
   (D) If Robert cannot ski on snow, he will not be able to ski on water.
   (E) The old man's dizziness must have been caused by pesticides in the water he drank from that stream.

4. Tears are seldom shed for the test examiner. Is he not some mythical monster, descendant of the Sphinx or Rumpelstiltskin, ready to tear apart any unsuspecting human being who fails to guess his riddles? Who would ever begin to recognize that kindly Professor, bumbling, absentminded, and generous to a fault, under that lion's skin? How could he have set such nasty questions; why didn't he tell us we ought to read up on Keats, when he had been holding forth on Shelley all year long?

   Which of the following can be deduced from the above?

   (A) What the professor has not lectured on will always turn up in the examination.
   (B) Rumpelstiltskin was the father of a mythical monster.
   (C) Examination questions, like riddles, need inspired guesses.
   (D) Nobody feels sorry for examiners.
   (E) Examination anxiety causes students to feel sorry for themselves.

5. Plato's political program leaned more on the institution rather than the individual, and he hoped to arrest political change by institutional control of succession in leadership. This control was to be educational, based upon an authoritarian view of learning, i.e., upon the authority of the learned expert and "the man of proven probity". This is how Plato interpreted Socrates' demand that a responsible politician should love truth and wisdom rather than exploit his expertise. The politician was deemed wise only if he knew his limitations.

   Which of these statements fits the text?

   (A) Plato's ideal society was essentially static.
   (B) Socrates supported Plato's notion of education by experts.
   (C) Plato advocated the imprisonment of political agitators.
   (D) Plato saw the need for teachers to be in control of government.
   (E) Socrates did not consider that experts were responsible enough to be politicians.

6. Whether or not there are fewer mental disorders in simpler non-Western cultures is difficult to judge, not only because of inadequate statistics, but also because behavior considered normal by our standards may be regarded by others as peculiar. Conversely, behavior considered abnormal in our society, e.g., trance, possession, and visionary experience, is perfectly acceptable in many other cultures. Furthermore, determining the rate of incidence of mental disorder can be complicated by "culturally patterned defects" in behavior which, although culturally approved, may be emotionally crippling.

   Which of the following can be deduced from the passage?

   (A) Mentally disturbed people in non-Western cultures act no differently from the sane.
   (B) Mental abnormality may be induced by social factors.
   (C) There cannot be statistical tables drawn up to cover abnormalities in non-Western cultures.
   (D) People who are emotionally retarded may be socially approved of in other societies.
   (E) Simple people of non-Western cultures can mistake our normal behavior for sexual deviance.

7. That man had progressed specifically by eliminating less effective human competitors, a kind of self-improvement of the of the human race, was a view supported by Social Darwinism. Self-help was made the fashion and tycoons were seen as the pillars of society. "Improvability" became an intellectual juggernaut transporting the full weight of the biological and social sciences.

   With which of the following would the author agree?

   (A) Darwinism sponsored social competitiveness.
   (B) Successful businessmen mark the highest level yet achieved by homo sapiens.
   (C) Biological survival is accompanied by improved social organization.
   (D) Darwin's theories showed the inevitability of human progress.
   (E) It is never possible to do things better than the way they are actually done.

Questions 8 — 9 are based on the following statements:

When John travels to an unfamiliar city, he will go to see a film only if there is no concert to attend. He always visits the local museum if there is one in the city, but he invariably goes to a film rather than visit a local scenic attraction. During a vacation trip to a region he had not visited before, John had a chance to spend a day in City X. John found out about all the events and activities in the city, but with time for only one holiday activity, he went to see a film.

8. Which of the following statements must have been true when John visited City X if the statements above are correct.

   (A) There was a concert in the City X.
   (B) There is a local museum in City X.
   (C) There is a local scenic attraction in City X.
   (D) There is no local museum in City X.
   (E) There is no local scenic attraction in City X.

9. John also spent a day in City Y and attended a baseball game. He knew about all events in City Y but went only to one activity.

   If the statements above are true, which of the following conclusions must also be true?

   (A) John prefers seeing a baseball game to visiting a local museum.
   (B) There is no local scenic attraction in City Y.
   (C) No concert was scheduled when John was in City Y.
   (D) There were no films playing in City Y.
   (E) There is no local museum in City Y.

10. The dim apprehension of some great principle can clothe itself with tremendous emotional force. In primitive times, particular actions arising out of such complex feelings were often brutish and nasty. Civilized language provides a whole group of words, each embodying the general idea under its own specialization, but to reach the common generality, the whole group of words must be gathered together with the hope of determining their common element, a procedure necessary for philosophical generalization.

    Which of the following can be deduced from this passage?

    (A) Intuitive responses tend to revert to primitive behavior.
    (B) We must study languages in order to understand philosophy.
    (C) The consideration of principles may be accompanied by vague fears which lead to emotional outbursts.
    (D) Strong emotion leads to violence.
    (E) Civilized language deals in particulars from which generalized concepts can be deduced.

11. Florence Nightingale recognised that men insisted that women should be happy, and that women therefore were required to assert that they were happy - regardless of their actual circumstances. Men took it as a personal affront if the women they "supported" complained of being unhappy. Consequently, women, who wished to continue to be supported, continued to claim to be happy even when most miserable.

    With which of the following would the author agree?

    (A) Women's happiness depended on their husbands' incomes.
    (B) Florence Nightingale cast serious doubt on the validity of women's testimony.
    (C) Married women claimed to be unhappy only to spite their husbands.
    (D) Women always say the opposite to what they actually mean.
    (E) Men and women have different ideas of what constitutes happiness.

12. An insurance firm requested quotations for a shipment of office paper and computer supplies. From the quotations received, it was clear that Acorn Supplies was more expensive that Barbery Stationers, and the prices from Landmark Office Suppliers were higher than those of Midland Papers Incorporated. Also, while the Midland Papers quotation was less than that received from Polygon Products, the figures received from Barbery Stationers and Polygon Products were so close to each other that there was no distinction between them.

    If the information is correct, which of the following must also be true?

    (A) The Landmark quotation must exceed that of Polygon Products.
    (B) Landmark prices are higher than prices at Acorn Supplies.
    (C) Barbery submitted a lower quotation than Landmark did.
    (D) Acorn's quotation ran higher than that of Midland Papers.
    (E) The Barbery quotation was below the quotation from Midland Papers.

13. The double invention known as printing, i.e., the development of typography for text and engraving for images, was the milestone marking the transition from the Middle Ages to the Renaissance. This event resulted not only from the genius of many scholars and men of science but also from the zeal and devotion of printers and publishers. The latter were not merely businessmen, as are most of their modern equivalents; they loved scholarship and science and many were scholars in their own right. They were in business, of course, and had to deal with business matters, as well.

With which of the following would the author agree?

(A) Renaissance businessmen had to be scholars to be successful.
(B) Printers and publishers were men of strong religious convictions.
(C) The development of printing required combined efforts of intellect and practical experience.
(D) Printers relieved scholars and scientists of their business worries.
(E) Printing was not known in the Middle Ages.

14. The way that laboratory rats learn their way through a maze provides important evidence against the notion that all animal learning is a building up of associative links. The evidence is that animals such as rats do not learn mazes by chains of conditioned responses and sub-goals, but rather that they build up internal "maps" of the maze, with the goal in the center as a focal point in their cognitive map.

Which of the following statements, if true, would tend to support the conclusion of the paragraph above?

(A) Rats tend to make a greater number of errors made towards, rather than away from, the center of the maze.
(B) Insects learn to find their way sequentially through a maze by building up from separate moves.
(C) Laboratory rats are cleverer than ordinary rats.
(D) Rats have shown themselves incapable of developing abstract systems to attain objectives.
(E) The training of circus dogs to do acrobatics proceeds by the presence of incentives.

15. Every schoolboy knows of the Eskimos; with their fuzzy fur garments, their round igloos and round bodies, they have come to symbolize winter and all it implies. In world history they stand out as the first people who, without firewood, could adapt themselves to (and even seem to enjoy) such extremes of climate. In Alaska the treeline lies far inland, and the Eskimos had to boil their food over stone or pottery lamps, using blubber as fuel.

Which of the following would be a likely explanation for the above?

(A) Eskimos prefer to use lamps for cooking rather than use the lamps to provide light.
(B) As firewood is a prime necessity for the development of sophisticated cooking techniques, Alaskan Eskimos live on a monotonous diet.
(C) In extremely cold climates, humans develop subcutaneous fat, and Eskimos are descended from peoples who lived in cold climates.
(D) Forests lie close to the shore in Siberia and the Siberian inhabitants were able to construct wood-frame tents and cook over wood fires.
(E) The ancestors of the Eskimo originally lived in a land that was much warmer than Alaska or Siberia is now.

16. Distinctive sounds come wrapped in an envelope of other disturbances of the air that convey such information as whether the speaker has a cold, is eating, feels angry, is a long way off or is an adult rather than a child. Only part of the sound wave corresponds to the central organization, a narrow and precisely limited set of contrasts between various combinations of pitches, durations, loudnesses, and voice and whisper, which are the audible results of the variety of ways we use our speech organs.

    Each of the following statements is consistent with the above paragraph EXCEPT

    (A) Sounds which carry meaning do not need to be separated out from those which give extraneous information about the speaker.
    (B) We may not understand what is being said if the speaker has his mouth full of food.
    (C) It is not possible to explore the central organization of the vocal system by singing scales.
    (D) Sounds that come from a distance can lose their central organization because of external effects such as the wind.
    (E) The internal organization of sound waves is very complex.

17. The Astra Pen is a newly-marketed disposable pen which can be used for an average of three years without running out of ink. The rapid growth of its pen sales in the last four years has seen a corresponding growth in profits for Star Products, the manufacturer. The managing director of Star Products is certain that a major increase in the production levels of Astra Pens would increase the growth of the profits of the company still further.

    Each of the following, if true, would weaken the conclusion drawn above EXCEPT

    (A) Two other pen manufacturers are expected to launch similar versions of the Astra Pen within the next four months.
    (B) Increased production levels cannot be achieved unless additional manufacturing equipment is purchased.
    (C) Increased production levels would justify converting all production to the use of new materials with marked reductions in the material unit costs.
    (D) Marketing research carried out by Star Products suggests that most sales last year were to Astra pen owners replacing their original pen.
    (E) Since the Astra Pen tends to be a seasonal purchase and stocks have to be stockpiled to meet peak demand, increased storage facilities will have to be purchased as current storage facilities are being used to capacity.

18. Sight has generally been regarded as our main source of knowledge of the world of objects, though requiring the sense of touch as a back-up and check. This would suggest that vision is regarded as comparatively "indirect"; that we can touch reality, while for vision we are linked to things that we see by light. This link has always been mysterious. It may be broken by darkness; it may bend or disperse to distort and mislead.

    Which of the following would be a logical extension of the above?

    (A) "I see" is often used to mean "I understand".
    (B) If we can touch things we can prove that they are there.
    (C) What we make out in partial darkness must be misleading.
    (D) We do not see things clearly if we look at them straight on.
    (E) In poor light we can see things that are not there.

19. At the very roots of Chinese thinking and feeling lies the principle of polarity, which is not be confused with the ideas of opposition or conflict. In the metaphors of other cultures, light is at war with darkness, life with death, good with evil, and the positive with the negative, and thus an idealism to cultivate the former and seek to eliminate the latter flourishes throughout most of the world. To the traditional way of Chinese thinking, this is as incomprehensible as an electric current without both positive and negative poles, for polarity is the principle that plus and minus, north and south, are different aspects of one and the same system.

    With which of the following statements would the author most likely agree?

    (A) Chinese philosophers have succeeded in resolving ideological conflicts.
    (B) Non-Chinese cultures tend to explain human history in dualistic terms.
    (C) The Chinese do not need a moral code.
    (D) Polarization causes good and evil to be considered irreconcilable opposites.
    (E) Chinese philosophers would not be able to understand how an electric current works.

20. Generally, most American Indians had respect, if not reverence and awe, for the earth and for all of nature, and, living close to nature and its forces, strove to exist in balance with them. If harmony with nature were disturbed, it was thought that illness, pain, death or other misfortunes would result. To most Indians, life after death was regarded as a continuation of existence in another world. Few thought of it, however, specifically as a hunter's paradise. The expression "happy hunting ground", (a white man's invention), merely symbolized the belief of some Indians that it was a good land where everything, including the securing of food, was easier for people than it had been before.

    Which of the following, if true, would cast doubt on the general theme suggested in the statements above?

    (A) American Indians used herbal medicines.
    (B) Totem poles were intended to be monuments to the dead.
    (C) American Indians killed for sport.
    (D) Initially, the American Indian welcomed the arrival of the white man.
    (E) American Indians believed that animals also would have life after death.

STOP

YOU MAY CHECK YOUR WORK ON THIS SECTION ONLY UNTIL YOUR TIME IS UP.
DO NOT WORK ON ANY OTHER SECTION.

SECTION IV

Time - 30 minutes

25 Questions

Directions: Each of the data sufficiency problems below consists of a question and two statements, labeled (1) and (2), in which certain data are given. You have to decide whether the data given in the statements are sufficient for answering the question. Using the data given in the statements plus your knowledge of mathematics and everyday facts (such as the number of days in July or the meaning of counterclockwise), you are to blacken space

- A if statement (1) ALONE is sufficient, but statement (2) alone is not sufficient to answer the question asked;
- B if statement (2) ALONE is sufficient, but statement (1) alone is not sufficient to answer the question asked;
- C if BOTH statements (1) and (2) TOGETHER are sufficient to answer the the question asked, but NEITHER statement ALONE is sufficient;
- D if EACH statement ALONE is sufficient to answer the question asked;
- E if statements (1) and (2) TOGETHER are NOT sufficient to answer the question asked, and additional data specific to the problem are needed.

Numbers: All numbers used are real numbers.

Figures: A figure in a data sufficiency problem will conform to the information given in the question, but will not necessarily conform to the additional information given in statements (1) and (2).

You may assume that lines shown as straight are straight and that angle measures are greater than zero.

You may assume that the position of points, angles, regions, etc., exist in the order shown.

All figures lie in a plane unless otherwise indicated.

Examples:

In triangle PQR, what is the value of x?

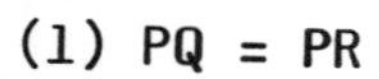
(1) PQ = PR

(2) y = 40

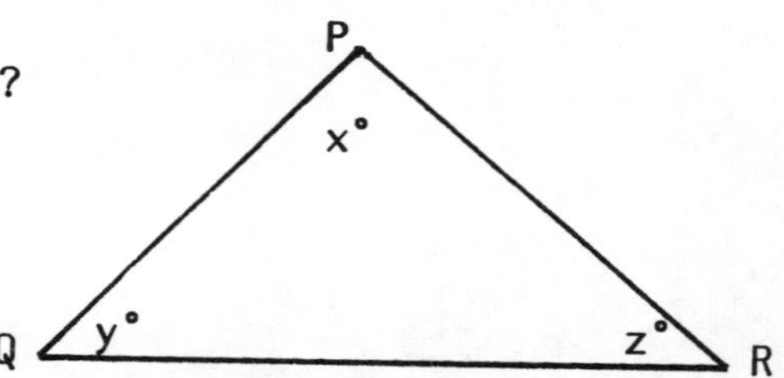

Explanation: According to statement (1), PQ = PR; therefore, triangle PQR is isosceles and y = z. Since x+y+z = 180, x+2y = 180. Since statement (1) does not give a value for y, you cannot answer the question using statement (1) by itself. According to statement (2), y = 40; therefore, x+z = 140. Since statement (2) does not give a value for z, you cannot answer the question using statement (2) by itself. Using both statements together, you can find y and z; therefore, you can find x, and the answer to the problem is C.

GO ON TO THE NEXT PAGE

A Statement (1) ALONE is sufficient, but statement (2) alone is not sufficient.
B Statement (2) ALONE is sufficient, but statement (1) alone is not sufficient.
C BOTH statements TOGETHER are sufficient, but NEITHER statement alone is sufficient.
D EACH statement ALONE is sufficient.
E Statements (1) and (2) TOGETHER are NOT sufficient.

1. A suit in a sale is reduced in price by 25%. At the end of the sale, the price of the suit is increased by 20% of the sale price. In dollars, what was the difference in price, before and after the sale?

   (1) The price after the sale was 90% of the price before the sale.

   (2) The sale price was $225.

2. Mr. Jones is employed as a salesman and earns 2% commission on all sales he makes in addition to a weekly salary of $270. What was his average weekly sales in February?

   (1) In February, Mr. Jones' weekly income averaged $318.

   (2) Jones averaged $48 per week in commissions during February.

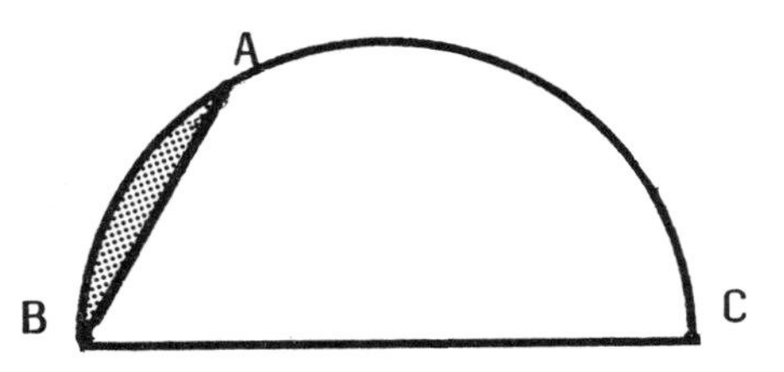

3. In the figure above, BC is a diameter. What is the area of the shaded region?

   (1) The arc BAC is 10π centimeters in length.

   (2) Angle ABC is 60°

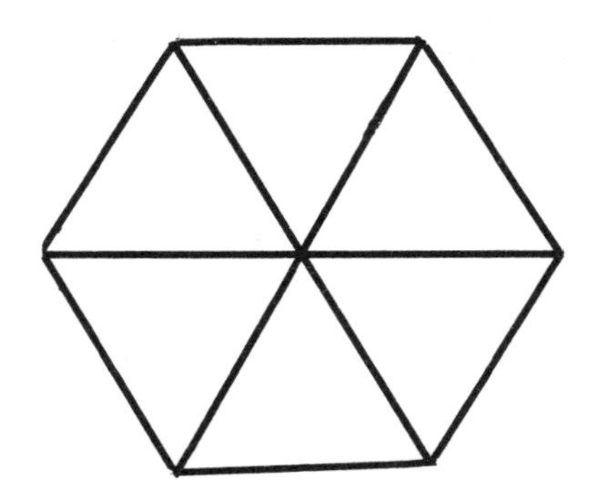

4. A window in the shape of a hexagon is made up of six identically shaped panes of glass. What is the area of the window?

   (1) The area of each pane is $\sqrt{3}$ square meters.

   (2) The perimeter of the hexagon is exactly 12 meters.

5. A piece of machinery depreciates by 20% of its current value each year. What was the original cost of the machinery?

   (1) The machinery was purchased exactly 3 years ago and now its value is $5,120.

   (2) Two years after the machinery was bought, its depreciated value was 64% of its cost.

GO ON TO THE NEXT PAGE

A Statement (1) ALONE is sufficient, but statement (2) alone is not sufficient.
B Statement (2) ALONE is sufficient, but statement (1) alone is not sufficient.
C BOTH statements TOGETHER are sufficient, but NEITHER statement alone is sufficient.
D EACH statement ALONE is sufficient.
E Statements (1) and (2) TOGETHER are NOT sufficient.

6. A magazine, currently sold on the newsstand at $2 per copy is to have the newsstand price increased 50%. What will be the percentage increase in revenue from the new price on the newsstands?

(1) At the original price, 30,000 copies are sold on newsstands.

(2) For every $0.25 increase in price, there is a reduction of 5% in the numbers sold on the newsstands.

7. If $x^2 + ax + b = (x + r)^2$, what is the value of r?

(1) b = 9

(2) a = - 6

	A	B
Dried Fruits	25%	60%
Nuts	40%	20%

8. A mixture of dried fruits, nuts and candy is to be made by combining mixtures A and B, which have dried fruits and nuts in the proportions shown in the table above. How many pounds of mixture A is needed for 100 pounds of the new mixture?

(1) The new mixture has 39 pounds of dried fruits.

(2) Candy represents 35% of mixture A and 20% of mixture B

9. In a manufacturing plant, a machine needed to manufacture steel bolts costs a fixed amount for set-up and overhead costs. If labor and materials cost $0.033 per bolt in lots of 1000 bolts, how large a production run is needed to cover the cost of making these bolts?

(1) A box of these bolts sells to wholesalers at a profit of 12%.

(2) An order of 100,000 bolts costs $3,300 for labor and materials.

10. Mr. Smith bought a house on which he obtained a mortgage for 90% of the price of the house. When the mortgage is paid off, will the total interest paid exceed the amount of the original mortgage?

(1) The interest rate is fixed at 10% simple interest per year.

(2) The mortgage will be paid off by 300 equal monthly payments.

GO ON TO THE NEXT PAGE

A Statement (1) ALONE is sufficient, but statement (2) alone is not sufficient.
B Statement (2) ALONE is sufficient, but statement (1) alone is not sufficient.
C BOTH statements TOGETHER are sufficient, but NEITHER statement alone is sufficient.
D EACH statement ALONE is sufficient.
E Statements (1) and (2) TOGETHER are NOT sufficient.

11. The digits from 0 to 9 can be represented by a different letter of the alphabet in a certain code. If each letter always represents the same digit and the sum

```
  B O B
+ T O M
-------
B I L L
```

is correct when expressed in digits, what is the digit represented by M?

(1) The letter O represents 7.

(2) The letter L represents 4.

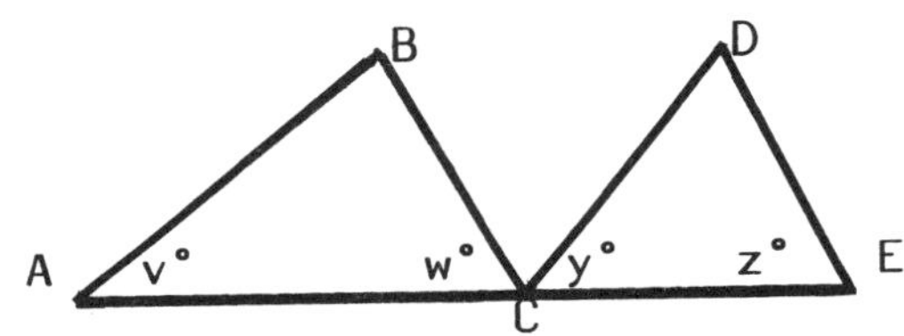

12. In the figure above, BC ∥ DE. What is the value of $y + z$?

(1) AB ∥ CD.

(2) AB = BC = AC.

13. What is the value of $x + y$?

(1) $3x + 5y = 41$

(2) $21x + 35y = 287$

14. Andy, Betty, and Carol are in a mathematics contest. Who had the highest score?

(1) The difference between Betty's score and Carol's is 6 points.

(2) Andy had a lower score than Betty.

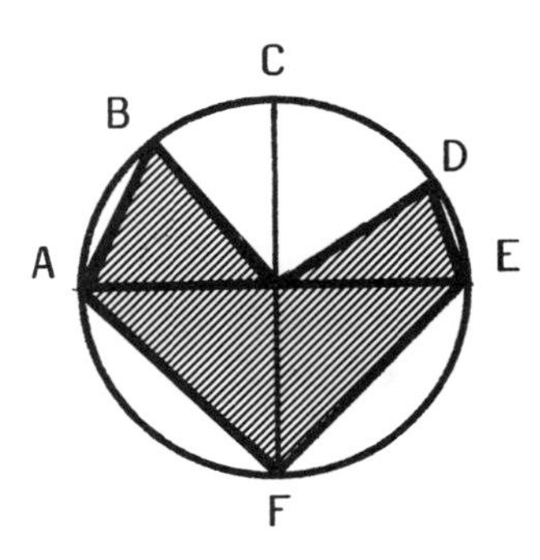

15. The shaded region shown above is inscribed in a circle with center, O, and diameters AE and CF. If the radius is 4, what is the area of the shaded region?

(1) Angle DOE = 60°

(2) The shaded region is symmetrical about CF.

16. If S is the sum of six different prime numbers, is S an odd number?

(1) The sum of two of the numbers is an odd number.

(2) Only three of the numbers have more than two digits.

GO ON TO THE NEXT PAGE

A Statement (1) ALONE is sufficient, but statement (2) alone is not sufficient.
B Statement (2) ALONE is sufficient, but statement (1) alone is not sufficient.
C BOTH statements TOGETHER are sufficient, but NEITHER statement alone is sufficient.
D EACH statement ALONE is sufficient.
E Statements (1) and (2) TOGETHER are NOT sufficient.

17. Is the quadrilateral, ABCD, a square?

(1) The sides of ABCD all have the same length.

(2) The diagonals of ABCD are equal in length.

18. Of the four people in a group, John, Tom, Mary, and Frank, Tom is taller than John, and Mary is shorter than Tom. Is Frank taller than Tom?

(1) Frank is shorter than John.

(2) Frank is taller than one person.

19. When the integer, M, is divided by 4, the remainder is 1. What is the value of M?

(1) When M + 3 is divided by 5, the result is an integer greater than 6 but less than 9.

(2) M is a prime number between 15 and 60 and M − 1 is a multiple of 3.

20. If x is an integer, is the average (arithmetic mean) of 65, 66, x, 70, and 71 equal to 68?

(1) x is the average of four of the numbers.

(2) $\frac{65 + x + 71}{3} = x$

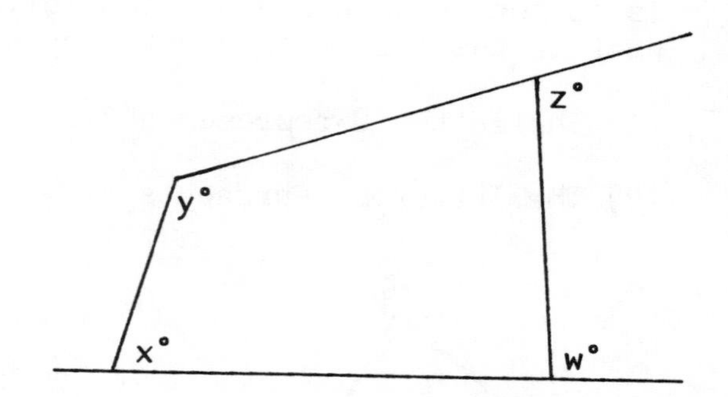

21. For the figure above, what is the value of z?

(1) $x = 60$

(2) $y = w$

GO ON TO THE NEXT PAGE

A Statement (1) ALONE is sufficient, but statement (2) alone is not sufficient.
B Statement (2) ALONE is sufficient, but statement (1) alone is not sufficient.
C BOTH statements TOGETHER are sufficient, but NEITHER statement alone is sufficient.
D EACH statement ALONE is sufficient.
E Statements (1) and (2) TOGETHER are NOT sufficient.

22. If w, x, y, and z are numbers such that the square of x plus the square of y exceeds, by 1, the cube of w plus the square of z, what is the value of w?

(1) $x^2 - z^2 = 12$ and $y = 4$

(2) $x = y = 4$

23. If $x^2 - 2xy - 2wx + 2xz = z^3$, and w, x, y, and z are integers, what is the value of x?

(1) $z = w + y$

(2) $z = 4$

24. If $x + y \neq 0$, how large is $\frac{(x + y)^2}{x^2 - y^2}$?

(1) $x + y = 7$

(2) $x - y = \frac{(x + y)}{7}$

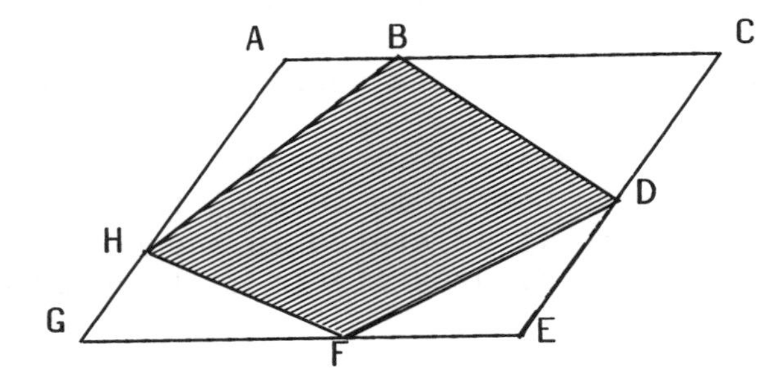

25. What is the area of the shaded region above?

(1) ACEG has an area of 64, and AB = CD = EF = GH.

(2) The area of BCD is 6.

S T O P

YOU MAY CHECK YOUR WORK ON THIS SECTION ONLY UNTIL YOUR TIME IS UP.
DO NOT WORK ON ANY OTHER SECTION.

SECTION V

Time - 30 minutes

20 Questions

Directions: In this section solve each problem, using any available space on the page for scratchwork. Then indicate the best answer of the answer choices given.

Numbers: All numbers used are real numbers.

Figures: Figures that accompany problems in this text are intended to provide information useful in solving the problem. They are drawn as accurately as possible EXCEPT when it is stated in a specific problem that its figure is not drawn to scale. All figures lie in a plane unless otherwise indicated.

1. A retailer sells a radio with a 20% rebate based on the manufacturer's recommended retail price (MRRP). If, in addition, the retailer gives a 15% discount on the MRRP, what is the final net cost to a customer who buys a radio with a MRRP of $15 ?

(A) $13.25
(B) $10.25
(C) $9.75
(D) $5.25
(E) $4.80

2. If a taxicab costs $2.25 for the first $\frac{1}{4}$ mile and $0.50 for each $\frac{1}{4}$ mile thereafter, what is the taxi fare for a trip of $4\frac{1}{2}$ miles?

(A) $11.25
(B) $10.75
(C) $10.00
(D) $6.75
(E) $2.75

3. Which of the following = $(\sqrt{6} - \sqrt{2})^2$?

(A) $2 - \sqrt{3}$ (C) 2 (E) $3 - \sqrt{3}$

(D) $6 - 3\sqrt{6}$ (E) $8 - 4\sqrt{3}$

4. If $x + y = 6(x - y)$ and $x \neq y$,

then $\dfrac{x^2 - y^2}{2(x - y)^2} =$

(A) 12 (B) 6 (C) 4

(D) 3 (E) $\frac{3}{4}$

GO ON TO THE NEXT PAGE

5. 8.047 - 1.69 =

(A) 7.643
(B) 6.357
(C) 5.498
(D) 5.358
(E) 5.022

6. Mr. Franklin bought 50 shares of stock in Company X for $75 per share. A year later, the stock was split 2 for 1 and six months after that, Company X issued a further 10% stock dividend. If Mr. Franklin sells his shares at $80 per share, what will be his net gain on the transactions?

(A) $375
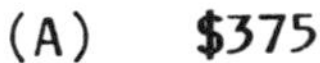
(B) $3,750
(C) $5,050
(D) $8,000
(E) $8,800

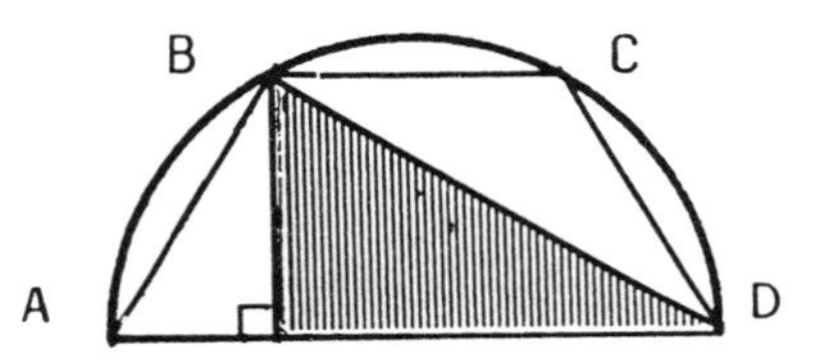

7. The four-sided figure, ABCD, is inscribed in a semi-circle as shown above. If AB = BC = CD, then the area of the shaded triangle is what fraction of the area of ABCD?

(A) $\frac{1}{2}$ (B) $\frac{4}{7}$ (C) $\frac{5}{8}$

(D) $\frac{3}{4}$ (E) $\frac{11}{18}$

8. If a, b, and c are consecutive integers greater than 15, and two of these have only one divisor other than 1, then the sum of a + c can always be divided by

(A) 8
(B) 9
(C) 10
(D) 11
(E) 12

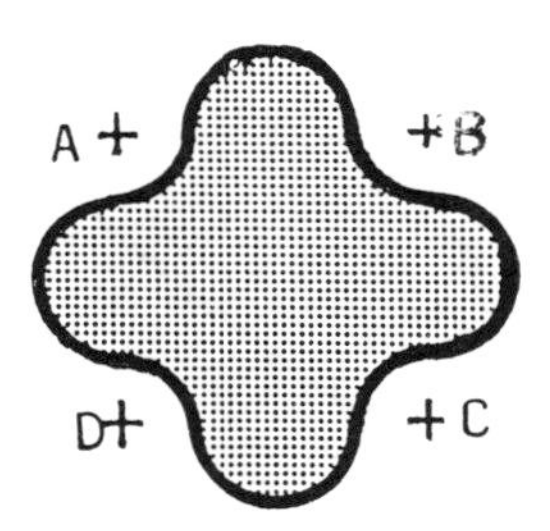

9. A design for a concrete pillar has a cross-section consisting of quarter circles and semi-circles as shown. If the points, A, B, C, and D are the centers from which the quarter circles are drawn, and these points are 8 centimeters apart, what is the perimeter of the cross-section in centimeters?

(A) 3π (B) 4π (C) 6π (D) 9π (E) 12π

GO ON TO THE NEXT PAGE

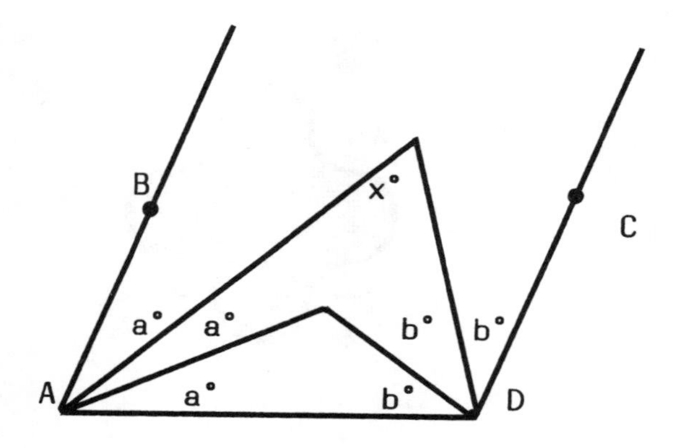

10. In the figure above, what is the value of x if AB ∥ CD?

(A) 45
(B) 60
(C) 90
(D) 120
(E) 150

11. The average of five consecutive numbers is 87. If each of the original numbers is reduced by 2 and then divided by 5, the average of the final set of numbers is

(A) 14.4
(B) 15.2
(C) 16.4
(D) 17.0
(E) 18.5

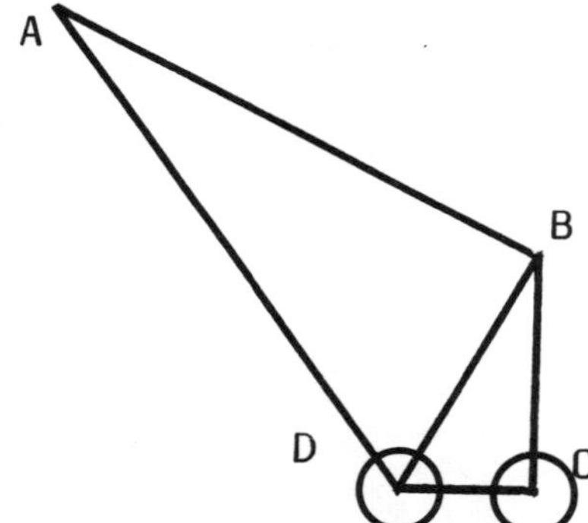

12. The design for a crane has a side view in the form of two right triangles as shown above. If the lengths, AB = 3BC = 4DC, and DC is 3 meters long, how long is the boom of the crane, AD?

(A) 8 (B) 11 (C) 13 (D) $14\frac{1}{2}$ (E) 17

13. A set of numbers is formed using a rule that the nth term is equal to $4n^2 + 1$, for all positive n. In this set, the difference in value between the nth term and the next larger term is

(A) 4 (B) 12 (C) $3n^2$ (D) $8n + 4$ (E) $8 + n^2$

14. The management of a store holding a 4-week sale finds that the average of daily sales increases each week by the same amount. If the overall average for the entire sale was $3,300 and the average for week 3 was 20% higher than the average for week 2, by how much did the average for the last week exceed the average daily sales for the first week?

(A) $1,320
(B) $1,800
(C) $1,920
(D) $2,640
(E) $3,960

15. If n* is equal to $\frac{(n-2)(n)(n+2)}{4}$

then the value of $\frac{12^*}{5^*}$ is

(A) 12.0
(B) 12.8
(C) 14.0
(D) 14.3
(E) 16.0

16. A set of 17 consecutive integers has an average value, M. A new set is constructed by adding 20 to the smallest number, 19 to the next, 18 to the third, etc. If the average of the new set is N, then N − M =

(A) 16 (B) 14 (C) 12 (D) 10 (E) 8

GO ON TO THE NEXT PAGE

17. Which of the following is correctly listed in order of <u>increasing</u> value?

(A) $2^{\frac{3}{4}}$, $3^{\frac{1}{2}}$, $4^{\frac{1}{4}}$

(B) $2^{\frac{3}{4}}$, $4^{\frac{1}{4}}$, $3^{\frac{1}{2}}$

(C) $4^{\frac{1}{4}}$, $3^{\frac{1}{2}}$, $2^{\frac{3}{4}}$

(D) $4^{\frac{1}{4}}$, $2^{\frac{3}{4}}$, $3^{\frac{1}{2}}$

(E) $3^{\frac{1}{2}}$, $4^{\frac{1}{4}}$, $2^{\frac{3}{4}}$

18. If x and y are positive integers such that

$\frac{1}{3} > \frac{1}{x + 3} > \frac{1}{9}$ and $2 < y^2 < 20$

which of the following could <u>not</u> be correct?

(A) $x < 5y^2$ (B) $y^2 < x$ (C) $2x < y$

(D) $2x + 9y < 2y^2$ (E) $x^2 + y^2 = 25$

19. If $S = \frac{1}{3} - \frac{1}{4} + \frac{1}{5} - \frac{1}{6} + \frac{1}{7}$,

then the value of S must be

(A) less than 0

(B) between 0 and $\frac{1}{7}$

(C) between $\frac{1}{7}$ and $\frac{1}{3}$

(D) between $\frac{1}{7}$ and $\frac{5}{7}$

(E) greater than $\frac{5}{7}$

20. If N = 1000X + 100Y + 10Z, where X, Y, and Z are different positive integers less than 4, the remainder when N is divided by 9 is

(A) 2 (B) 4 (C) 6 (D) 8

(E) a prime number

S T O P

YOU MAY CHECK YOUR WORK ON THIS SECTION ONLY UNTIL YOUR TIME IS UP.
DO NOT WORK ON ANY OTHER SECTION.

SECTION VI

Time — 30 minutes

25 Questions

Directions: In each of the following sentences, some part of the sentence or the entire sentence is underlined. Beneath each sentence you will find five ways of phrasing the underlined part. The first of these repeats the original; the other four are different. If you think the original is better than any of the alternatives, choose answer A; otherwise choose one of the others. Select the best version and blacken the corresponding space on your answer sheet.

This is a test of correctness and effectiveness of expression. In choosing answers, follow the requirements of standard written English; that is, pay attention to grammar, choice of words, and sentence construction. Choose the answer that expresses most effectively what is presented in the original sentence; this answer should be clear and exact, without awkwardness, ambiguity, or redundancy.

1. Neither the municipal assessors nor the mayor himself seem to have been aware of the city's failure to follow federal guidelines on the employment of women and ethnic minorities.

(A) nor the mayor himself seem
(B) or the mayor himself seems
(C) nor the mayor himself seems
(D) or the mayor himself seem
(E) or the mayor himself would seem

2. According to the university's department of psychology, the amount of paranormal phenomena reported to them has increased tenfold since the psychical research project began in 1968.

(A) amount of paranormal phenomena reported to them
(B) amount of paranormal phenomena reported to the department
(C) number of paranormal phenomena reported to it
(D) amount of paranormal phenomena reported to it
(E) number of paranormal phenomena reported to the department

3. Because it reacts explosively with water, metallic sodium is somewhat dangerous for high school chemistry students to handle.

(A) Because it reacts explosively with water, metallic sodium is
(B) Reacting explosively with water makes metallic sodium
(C) Inasmuch as it reacts explosively with water, metallic sodium is
(D) The fact of its reacting explosively with water makes metallic sodium
(E) Because it reacts explosively with water is why metallic sodium is

GO ON TO THE NEXT PAGE

4. In order to avoid delays in checking returned books, readers are asked by the librarian not to keep more than twelve volumes on their desk at a time, and to return each book as soon as it is no longer needed.

(A) readers are asked by the librarian not to keep more than twelve volumes on their desk
(B) readers are asked by the librarian not to keep more than twelve volumes on their desks
(C) readers are asked by the librarian to not keep more than twelve volumes on their desk
(D) the librarian asks readers not to keep more than twelve volumes on their desks
(E) the librarian asks readers to not keep more than twelve volumes on their desk

5. As with Hemingway, Mailer began his career as a novelist with a story about men's reactions to violence and death.

(A) As with Hemingway
(B) As had Hemingway
(C) Like Hemingway had
(D) Like Hemingway had done
(E) As had done Hemingway

6. Inasmuch as the oil speculation bubble had already burst, the cartel's decision to curtail expansion was the only logical one.

(A) Inasmuch as the oil speculation bubble had already burst
(B) Since the oil speculation bubble had already bust
(C) Being that the oil speculation bubble had already burst
(D) As the oil speculation bubble had already bursted
(E) Being as the oil speculation bubble had already bursted

7. Dissimilar to the tidal waves caused by hurricanes, the even more terrible tsunamis occur when an earthquake or volcano eruption on the ocean floor hurls a gigantic wave against Pacific coasts.

(A) Dissimilar to the tidal waves caused by hurricanes, the even more terrible tsunamis occur
(B) Unlike the tidal wave caused by a hurricane, the even more terrible tsunami is
(C) In contrast to the tidal wave caused by a hurricane, the even more terrible tsunami occurs
(D) Unlike the tidal waves caused by hurricanes, the even more terrible tsunamis are
(E) The even more terrible tsunami, unlike the tidal wave caused by a hurricane, is

GO ON TO THE NEXT PAGE

8. Although such action is not likely to gain it support, the faculty has decided to boycott this year's commencement exercises as a protest against low salaries.

(A) likely to gain it support, the faculty has
(B) liable to gain them support, the faculty have
(C) likely to gain them support, the faculty has
(D) liable to gain it support, the faculty has
(E) liable to gain it support, the faculty have

9. It is not surprising that neither of these nineteenth-century chemists appears to have realized the danger involved in the extraction of pure radium.

(A) It is not surprising that neither of these nineteenth-century chemists appears to have realized the danger involved in the extraction of pure radium.
(B) Neither of these nineteenth-century chemists appears, not surprisingly, to have realized the danger involved in the extraction of pure radium.
(C) Neither of these nineteenth-century chemists appears to have realized the danger involved in the extraction of pure radium, which is not surprising.
(D) Not surprisingly, neither of these nineteenth-century chemists appear to have realized the danger involved in the extraction of pure radium.
(E) Neither of these nineteenth-century chemists appear to have realized the danger involved in the extraction of pure radium, a fact which is not surprising.

10. According to a recent survey, many American university students are so uninterested in their studies that faculty members, exacerbated by this lack of intellectual curiosity, are increasingly leaving the teaching profession.

(A) uninterested in their studies that faculty members, exacerbated
(B) disinterested in their studies that faculty members, aggravated
(C) uninterested in their studies that faculty members, aggravated
(D) uninterested in their studies that faculty members, exasperated
(E) disinterested in their studies that faculty members, exasperated

11. Hardly to be prepared for a situation in which falling sales are accompanied by sharp increases in production costs, many small firms in the electronics industry are now facing bankruptcy.

(A) Hardly to be prepared for a situation in which
(B) Hardly prepared for a situation in which
(C) Hardly preparing for a situation where
(D) Hardly preparing for a situation in which
(E) Hardly prepared for a situation where

12. Although they are unable to publish it this year, the editors appreciate you sending them this masterfully researched article on superconductivity in cadmium.

(A) you sending them this masterfully
(B) that you have sent them this masterly
(C) it that you have sent them this masterfully
(D) you sending them this masterly
(E) your sending them this masterfully

GO ON TO THE NEXT PAGE

13. Ms. Pappas is one of the few Oklahoma state representatives who still is supporting the ratifying of both the Equal Rights Amendment and the proposed blue laws.

(A) is supporting the ratifying
(B) support ratification
(C) supports ratification
(D) supports ratifying
(E) support the ratifying

14. Because of the extra work and costs involved in sorting, processing, and mailing of international orders, the sales manager has directed that such orders be surcharged.

(A) sorting, processing, and mailing of
(B) the sorting of, processing of, and mailing of
(C) the sorting, processing, and mailing
(D) the sorting of, the processing of, and the mailing of
(E) sorting, processing, and mailing

15. Despite decades of remarkable progress in human paleontology, there is still much disagreement among physical anthropologists in regards to the genesis and lineal ancestry of "Homo sapiens."

(A) among physical anthropologists in regards to
(B) between physical anthropologists concerning
(C) between physical anthropologists with regards to
(D) among physical anthropologists with regard to
(E) among physical anthropologists about

16. That Blacks in the United States are increasingly joining the ranks of management and the professions does not mean they have, as a group, joined the mainstream of American society.

(A) That
(B) As
(C) In that
(D) Despite
(E) Because

17. The Mature Women's Studies Program was designed for women which either have been employed or have been housewives for at least ten years.

(A) which either have been employed or have
(B) who either have been employed or else
(C) which either have been employed or
(D) who have either been employed or
(E) either who have been employed or

GO ON TO THE NEXT PAGE

18. In the competition for the video, home computer, and leisure software markets, our competitors have so far been as successful as, if not more successful than, us.

(A) successful as, if not more successful than, us
(B) successful as, if not more successful than, we
(C) successful, if not more successful, than us
(D) successful as, if not more successful than, our efforts
(E) successful, if not more successful, than we

19. Isolated long enough, mutations along various lines in a species will begin, the inexplicable thing being the retention of traits having either no survival value or even a deleterious effect upon the organism.

(A) mutations along various lines in a species will begin, the inexplicable thing being the retention of
(B) a species will begin to mutate along various lines; but it is inexplicable that the species will retain
(C) a species' mutations along various lines will begin; but, inexplicably, the species will retain
(D) a species will begin to mutate along various lines, but inexplicably retaining
(E) a species will begin to mutate along various lines, the inexplicable thing being the retention of

20. Pater's emphases, many of which obviously derive after his appreciation of Pre-Raphaelite painting, may now seem intolerably mannered and impressionistic.

(A) many of which obviously derive after
(B) much of which obviously derives from
(C) many of which obviously derive from
(D) much of which obviously derives after
(E) of which much obviously derives from

21. The primary reason the substantial matriarchal contribution to the genesis of culture has been so little comprehended is because this has been distorted and obscured by the sexist orientation of historians and archeologists.

(A) because this has
(B) because this contribution has
(C) that this contribution has
(D) because of its having
(E) that this has

22. In the final competition between the gymnasts, Ms. Wong was adjudged to have had the more perfect form.

(A) had the more
(B) had the more nearly
(C) the most nearly
(D) had the most
(E) the more nearly

GO ON TO THE NEXT PAGE

23. Despite the conquest of the Roman Empire by Germanic people in the fifth century, Latin was even spoken in the German emperor's court, remaining the language of government, religion, and learning for centuries to come.

(A) Latin was even spoken in the German emperor's court, remaining
(B) Latin was even spoken in the German emperor's court, and it remained
(C) Latin, and it was even spoken in the German emperor's court, remained
(D) spoken even in the German emperor's court, Latin remained
(E) Latin, which was spoken even in the German emperor's court, remained

24. The candidate for mayor pledged to end corruption in city hall and that property and road taxes would not be raised.

(A) to end corruption in city hall
(B) an end to corruption in city hall
(C) that an end would come to corruption in city hall
(D) that city hall corruption was to be ending
(E) that corruption in city hall would be ended

25. If this case was being tried three hundred years ago, the defendant could demand not only that he vindicates himself by combat, but also that he sits higher in court than the plaintiff.

(A) was being tried three hundred years ago, the defendant could demand not only that he vindicates himself by combat, but also that he sits
(B) was being tried three hundred years ago, the defendant not only could have demanded that he vindicate himself by combat, but also that he sit
(C) were being tried three hundred years ago, the defendant could demand not only that he vindicates himself by combat, but also that he sits
(D) were being tried three hundred years ago, the defendant could demand not only that he vindicate himself by combat, but also that he sit
(E) were being tried three hundred years ago, the defendant not only could have demanded that he vindicate himself by combat, but also that he sit

End of Examination

STOP

YOU MAY CHECK YOUR WORK ON THIS SECTION ONLY UNTIL YOUR TIME IS UP.
DO NOT WORK ON ANY OTHER SECTION.

<u>Answers to the Second Examination</u>

	Section I	Section II	Section III	Section IV	Section V	Section VI
1.	E	C	D	B	C	C
2.	B	B	B	D	B	E
3.	E	A	C	C	E	A
4.	A	C	E	D	D	D
5.	C	D	A	A	B	B
6.	A	B	B	B	C	A
7.	A	E	A	B	A	C
8.	D	C	D	A	E	A
9.	B	C	E	E	E	A
10.	C	D	E	C	B	D
11.	D	A	B	D	D	B
12.	A	E	D	C	C	E
13.	E	D	C	E	D	B
14.	D	E	A	E	B	E
15.	C	A	B	C	E	E
16.	A	D	A	A	C	A
17.	B	A	C	C	D	D
18.	D	E	A	A	D	B
19.	E	B	B	D	C	B
20.	C	B	C	B	C	C
21.	B			C		C
22.	A			A		B
23.	D			E		E
24.	E			B		E
25.	B			E		D

Second Examination: Explanation of the Answers

Section I: Reading Comprehension.

1. Choice E best reflects the content and emphasis of the passage.

2. The correct answer, B, is neither stated nor implied in the first paragraph.

3. The correct answer, E, rather abruptly changes the subject, interrupting the sequence of thought in the paragraph.

4. The correct answer, A, includes I, which is answered in lines 6-9; II, which is answered in lines 26-29; and III, which is answered in line 43.

5. The correct answer, C, may be inferred from the context, as well as from the denotation of the words making up the phrase.

6. The correct answer, A, is explicitly stated in lines 20-22.

7. The correct answer, A, is contradicted by lines 26-29, which indicate that tyrosine is not an enzyme.

8. The correct answer, D, is the best inference from the last paragraph.

9. Choice B best reflects the content and the pattern of exposition of the passage.

10. The correct answer, C, best fits the author's style and organization. None of the other answer choices is borne out in the development of the passage.

11. The correct answer, D, includes only I, which is answered in lines 5-10.

12. The correct answer, A, may be gathered from the immediate context, as well as from the denotation of reified.

13. The correct answer, E, may be inferred from lines 8-12. The other answer choices fit the discussion of role in lines 13-28.

14. The correct answer, D, best reflects the author's tone, for example, in lines 1-5. This tone is that of a candid and helpful lecturer.

15. The correct answer, C, may be inferred from lines 8-17. The other answer choices are either contradicted or not supported by the passage.

16. The correct answer, A, is best supported by the immediate context, as well as by the discussion throughout the passage. Choice B may be ruled out by the phrase "any given situation," which includes more than role behavior. Similarly, the phrase "antecedent conditions" in choice E is too inclusive.

17. Choice B best reflects the emphasis of the passage.

18. The correct answer, D, may be gathered from the denotation of dystopian, as well as from the context. B may seem attractive, but it is less precise.

19. The correct answer, E, includes only I, which may be inferred from lines 2-3. II is neither stated nor implied in the passage; III may be ruled out by "turgid style," since Donnelly's style is not so characterized; and IV confuses Donnelly's point of view with that of Hofstadter.

20. The correct answer, C, is the best analogy with the kind of analysis emphasized by the author.

21. The correct answer, B, is contradicted by the implications of lines 34-39. In B, there is a confusion of the points of view of Donnelly and Hofstadter.

22. The correct answer, A, may be inferred from lines 14-31 taken together with the denotation of the expression, "a Jeremiah."

23. The correct answer, D, may be inferred by juxtaposing lines 21-29 and lines 31-34.

24. The correct answer, E, is indicated by the context, as well as by the denotation of apocalyptic. Choice C may seem attractive, but it may be ruled out by the emphasis of the context, as well as by the word symbolically, an ascription which is not justified by the passage.

25. The best answer, B, is strongly implied by lines 26-29. This inference is reinforced by lines 11-13 when taken together with the whole discussion of Donnelly's novel. D is less strongly implied.

Section II: Problem Solving.

1. In order to change 4 rows of 9 trees into 6 rows of 6 trees, then 12 trees, i.e., 3 trees from each of the original 4 rows, have to be replanted: choice C.

2. The expression can be rewritten as $(wx^3y^5z^7)(w^{-7}x^{-5}y^{-3}z^{-1})$, an expression that simplifies to $w^{-6}x^{-2}y^2z^6$, an equivalent form to choice B.

3. The decimals can be rewritten as $(3/8 \times 5/2 \times 4) \div (3 \times \frac{1}{2} \times \frac{1}{2})$ which simplifies to 5, choice A.

4. If a, b, and c are consecutive, one of these numbers must be a multiple of 2 and one must be a multiple of 3. Therefore, the product must be a multiple of 2 x 3 or 6, choice C.

5. Cancellation of common factors in the numerators and denominators reduces the expression to $k/7 = 1$, so k must equal 7, choice D.

6. Since triangle ABC is isosceles, AC = CB. Since the area is 72, then AC = 12. With this value and AD = 5, $CD^2 = 12^2 + 5^2$, from which CD = 13, choice B.

7. Replacing x with 0 gives $0 * y = (-y)^2/y^2 = y^2/y^2 = 1$ and I is correct. Since the expression $(x - y)^2 = (y - x)^2$, the order in which numbers are assigned does not affect the results, so II is correct. Using 1/y in the definition gives $(x - [1/y])^2/(x + [1/y])^2 = ([xy - 1]/y)^2/([xy + 1]/y)^2 = (xy - 1)^2/(xy + 1)^2 = [(xy - 1)/x]^2/[(xy + 1)/x]^2 = (y - [1/x])^2/(y + [1/x])^2 = y*(1/x)$. But because II is true, $y*(1/x) = (1/x)*y$, and therefore III is true. The correct choice is E.

8. Since a(ax) is a^2x, the maximum range is the result using $a^2 = 0$, $x = 3$, for the lowest value, and $a = -4$, $x = 7$, for the highest value, which gives choice C.

9. The distances between the successive intersections of the six semi-circles are, not only diameters of the semi-circles, but also equal to R, the radius from the center, C. Consequently, the perimeter is $\frac{1}{2}(\pi R)(6)$ which gives choice C.

10. Monthly sales are (15)($4,200) = $63,000 and commissions are received on $63,000 - $25,000 = $38,000. His commissions are 7½% of $38,000 = $2,850 monthly, $34,200 per year. Added to the annual salary, ($22,000), gives $56,200, choice D.

11. The capacity of the tank and barrel, respectively, are $\frac{1}{2}[\frac{1}{4}\pi D^2 L]$ and $\frac{1}{4}\pi(2D)^2 h$ where D and L are the diameter and length of the tank and 2D and h are its diameter and height of water in the barrel. If the tank was full, equating these two expressions would give: $h = L/8 = 480/8 = 60$ cm. As the tank is only 2/3 full, the water in the barrel rises to a level only 2/3 as high or 40 cm., choice A.

12. Equating the two expressions gives $y^2 + 6 - 5y = 12 - 7y + y^2$, from which $6 - 5y = 12 - 7y$, or $2y = 6$ and $y = 3$, choice E.

13. Since $AC^2 = 5^2 + 12^2$, then $AC = 13$. The area of this triangle is $\frac{1}{2}(12)5$ and this value must also equal $\frac{1}{2}(BD)(AC)$; $BD = 5(12)/13 = 60/13$, choice D.

14. From the statement of the problem, N can be expressed as $N = 8k + 4$, where k is any integer. If used in each of the choices suggested in turn, this expression gives: $8k + 6$; $48k + 9,876,567$; $24k + 33$; $4k + 3$; and $6k + 6$. Of these, only choice E will always be a multiple of 6, regardless of the value of k.

15. Since the ratio of a semi-circle to its diameter is $\frac{1}{2}\pi$, it follows that the ratio of perimeter of the figure to the perimeter of the triangle has the same value. The correct choice is A.

16. The first and third terms, combined and rewritten, give $\frac{1}{4}(x^2 + 2xy + y^2)$ which equals $\frac{1}{4}(x + y)^2$; this result combined with the second term gives $-\frac{1}{4}(x + y)^2$. The correct choice is D.

17. As all sides of this rhombus are equal, setting the expression for AB equal to the expression for AC produces: $-4x + 12 = -x$, from which $x = 4$. The simplest expression to evaluate is BC, which gives 12 as the length, choice A.

18. The average of 64, 65, 66 is 65, while the average of 11, 12, 13, 14, 15 is 13. The ratio of 65 to 13 is 5, choice E.

19. If every other piece is colored then six must be colored and six are not. The fraction colored must be 6/12 or ½. With a diameter of 12, the radius is 6 and the area is 36π. The shaded portion is half this value or 18π, choice B.

20. If V represents the original volume, and X amount of pure alcohol is added, then total alcohol present is $0.1V + X$ and this represents 25% of $V + X$. As an equation, this is: $0.1V + X = 0.25(V + X)$ which simplifies to $0.75X = 0.15V$. From this, the ratio, X/V is 1/5 or 20%, choice B.

Section III: Critical Reasoning.

1. The correct choice is D. The reason that scientists avoid value judgements is that these are only partly objective. Since linguists work by scientific techniques, the meaning of culture is confined to basic social structures, and not extended to the more evaluative, subjective sense that culture would have in non-scientific contexts.

2. The correct choice is B, which follows from "the ideas governing the erection of the stones must not have been static". As the construction of megalithic structures went on for a very long period, changing aspects of social developments would be reflected in the uses the stones were seen to provide - "... perhaps one scheme was ... replaced by another."

3. The best choice is C, which uses erroneous logic in the form: event B occurs after event A, therefore event B was caused by event A. There is no evidence presented to support the contentions that "eating peas" causes the "stomach ache", or that "soap" causes the "skin rash".

4. Choice E best reflects the tone of the passage where the ironic questions reflect the student's sense of injustice. The teacher or examiner could thus be blamed for the student's failure to review the course content properly.

5. Choice A is the best choice. The statement, " ... he hoped to arrest political change ... ", reflects this directly. Furthermore, "an authoritarian view of learning" would not allow for flexibility or innovation.

6. The correct choice, B, follows from the last sentence concerning ways that socially accepted behavior may cause emotional damage, thus causing aberrant mental processes.

7. The best choice is A. The last sentence suggests biology and sociology as the two sciences most affected by Darwin's theory of the "survival of the fittest," (paraphrased as "improvability" in the passage). Darwin's biological hypotheses were transferred readily to social contexts, where the survival of the fittest was easily understood in terms of material and psychological competitiveness.

8. Choice D is correct. The statements ranks leisure activities in the following order of decreasing preference: local museum, a concert, a film, a local scenic attraction. Of the choices offered, only D would fit these preferences.

9. The best answer is E. It is not known what preference is given to a baseball game in respect to a concert, a film, or a local scenic attraction. However, since the original statements imply that "visiting a museum" is an unconditional first preference, it follows that there is no museum to visit.

10. The correct choice is E, a paraphrase of the third sentence. Specialized terms are grouped according to some common factor, which can then be extracted to form a generalized concept. It is necessary to proceed from the particular to the general, not the other way round.

11. The best choice is B. The passage lists a number of reasons to doubt women's testimony since social and personal pressures required them to say they were happy whether this was true or not.

12. The correct choice is D. From the statements, Acorn's quotation is higher than Barbery which is equal to Polygon. Polygon is higher than Midland, so the Acorn quotation must be greater than th Midland quotation.

13. The correct choice is C. The development of printing required not only the intellectual inventiveness of "scholars and men of science" but also the practical expertise of the printers and publishers.

14. The correct choice is A. If, as the passage suggests, rats solve a maze using an internal "map", then, once experienced, it could be used to make the return journey more efficient. If, instead, learning was by associative links, the return path could be as complex as the journey toward the center.

15. Choice B is correct. As Alaskan Eskimos live far beyond the treeline, they have only rudimentary cooking facilities which would eliminate variety in food preparation.

16. The best choice is A. From the passage, "meaning" is carried only by the "central organization" and external factors need to be filtered out if communication is to be effective.

17. Choice C is the best choice. Increased profits can be guaranteed if either income is increased and/or unit costs are reduced. Choice A suggests a possible reduction in volume of sales with a corresponding reduction in income. Choices B and E both suggest the possibility of increased costs due to increase in production volume. Choice D suggests the possibility of a leveling off of demand (and correspondingly a leveling off of income) which would coincide with increased costs due to expanded production. Choice C alone, suggests the reduction in average costs with expanded production levels.

18. The correct choice is A. The first sentence suggests that functions of sight and understanding run so close together that they seem to be interchangeable.

19. The correct choice, B, paraphrases the second sentence of the passage, which suggests that non-Chinese cultures envisage a perpetual conflict between good and evil in human activities.

20. The best choice, C, would be the antithesis of the statements in the first sentence. It would not be possible to exhibit "respect, if not reverence and awe ... for all of nature ..." if the American Indian killed for sport.

Section IV: Data Sufficiency.

1. If X is the price before the sale, then the sale price is 0.75X and the post sale price is 1.2 times this latter value, i.e., 1.2(0.75X), or 0.9X. Statement (1) is simply a restatement of the consequence of the problem. With statement (2), setting 0.75X = 225 gives X = $300 and post-sale price of 0.9(300) = $270 gives answer to the problem, $30. The answer is B.

2. The answer is D. From statement (1), it follows that Jones made ($318 - $270) = $48 in commissions which represents $2,400 in sales. Using statement (2), the commissions received, $48, are given directly.

3. The answer is C. Using statement (1), the radius of the semicircle can be found to be 10, but no information is provided to work out the size of the sector, AB. Using (2), arc AC must represent 120° and arc AB must be 60°. The area of the sector is thus one-third the area of the semicircle less the area of an equilateral triangle with sides equal to the radius of the circle. Using (1) and (2) the answer is $50\pi/3 - 25\sqrt{3}$.

4. Choice D is the correct answer. Using the statement (1) the area is six times the area of the individual pane. Using statement (2), the length of one side of the equilateral triangles 12/6 = 2, and the area of one pane can be calculated to be the area given in statement (1).

5. In three years the value is reduced to (0.8)(0.8)(0.8) = 0.512 of its initial value. Using statement (1), the original value can be found to be $10,000. The second statement provides no absolute amount on which to compute initial costs. The best answer is A.

6. Using (1) alone, no information is available as to any changes in demand as a result of the price increase. From (2) it follows that for the $1 increase in price, the number of copies sold will be 20% fewer. For every 10 copies sold at the original price having a former revenue of $2 x 10 = $20, at the new price of $3, only 8 copies will be sold for a revenue of $3 x 8 = $24. From this the percentage increase in revenue is 100(24 - 20)/20 = 20%. The best answer is B.

7. Expansion of the right hand term and matching comparable terms gives rise to the expressions: $2r = a$, and $b = r^2$. Using statement (1) alone implies that r can be either + 3 or - 3. Using (2) alone gives r = - 3. The best answer is B.

8. Allowing A and B to represent the pounds of mixture A and B respectively in the new mixture it follows that A + B = 100, (from which B = 100 - A), the weight of dried fruit is equal to 0.25A + 0.60B, and the weight of nuts equals 0.40A + 0.20B. Using B = 100 - A in 0.25A + 0.60B = 39 from (1), gives 0.25A +0.6(100 - A) = 60 - 0.35A = 39 or 0.35A = 21, from which A = 60. Statement (2) gives no information beyond what could be deduced from the table of ingredients. The answer is A.

9. The answer is E. Neither (1) nor (2) provide information on set-up costs or overhead costs.

10. Neither (1) nor (2) give sufficient information to analyze the problem. Using the statements together, a simplified analysis will provide an answer. During the duration of the mortgage, the average amount outstanding on the mortgage is approximately ½ the initial value. On average, therefore, the yearly interest payments amount to 10% of the average mortgage value or 5% of the initial amount of the mortgage. In 25 years time, the approximate total interest payment will be approximately 25 x 5% or 125% of the mortgage. The best answer is C.

11. From the problem, it follows that B must stand for the digit, 1. If M is initially assumed to be 9, then, B + M = 1 + 9 = 10, and L must be zero. The next addition produces a contradiction, i.e., 0 + 0 + 1 = a sum with last digit, L, equal to zero. As 0 + 0 must be even, 0 + 0 + 1 must be odd and L would have to be an odd number; consequently, M is not 9, and L is not zero. With B + M less than 10, L must be an even digit since 0 + 0, an even sum, is a value with last digit, L. The value of L cannot be 2, however, since that would imply that M = 1, the same value as B and a contradiction of the problem statement that all letters represent different digits. Therefore, M must be 3, 5, or 7, depending on whether L is 4, 6, or 8. From statement (1), it follows that L must be 4 from which M = 3. From statement (2), it follows that M = 3, as before. The correct answer is D.

12. From the problem, w = z. From (1), it follows that v = y, but the value of y + z cannot be determined. Using (2) alone, triangle ABC is equilateral, v = w = z = 60°, but y + z cannot be evaluated. Using (1) and (2) together, it follows that y = 60° so y + z = 120°. The correct answer is C.

13. The correct answer is E. Statement (1) provides one equation in the two unknown quantities, x and y, which is insufficient. Statement (2) is equivalent to statement (1) multiplied by 7 and provides the same information as statement (1).

14. Statement (1) alone does not indicate which of the two scored higher. Statement (2) indicates that Betty's score was higher than Andy's but there is no way to rank Carol with the other two. The correct answer is E.

15. From the figure and the problem statement, the area of triangle AEF can be calculated as $\frac{1}{2}(4)(8) = 16$. From statement (1), it follows that triangle ODE is equilateral and as its sides must be 4, the area of this triangle can be determined. From statement (2) alone, the area of ABO must equal the area of triangle ODE but from this alone no values of areas can be determined. Using (1) and (2) together means that ABO is also an equilateral triangle with side 4 whose area is readily computed. The correct answer is C.

16. From statement (1), the two numbers that add up to an odd number must be 2 plus some other prime. This means that the six numbers include 2 plus five other prime numbers, the sum of which will always be an odd number. Using (2) alone, it follows that three of the numbers must be chosen from the numbers, 2, 3, 5, and 7. Since the answer rests on whether or not, one of the three chosen primes includes 2, this statement alone is not sufficient. The best answer is A.

17. Statement (1) alone implies that ABCD is a rhombus or a square. Statement (2) alone implies that ABCD is a rectangle, a square, or a symmetrical trapezoid (trapezium). Using both together requires ABCD to be a square. Answer is C.

18. The problem indicates that Tom is taller than both John and Mary but does not provide information on the relative heights of John, Mary, and Frank. From (1), Frank is shorter than Tom and the question is answered. Statement (2) alone only insures that Frank is taller than Mary or John, but there is no information as to the relative heights of Frank and Tom. The correct answer is A.

19. From the problem statement, it can be deduced that M must be an odd integer. From (1), $(M + 3)/5$ is either 7 or 8, i.e., M must be either 32 or 37, but since M is odd, M must equal 37. From the first part of (2), M must be 17, 29, 37, 41, or 53 because M must be 1 greater than some multiple of 4. Of these, only 37 is a number that is one greater than a multiple of 3. The correct answer is D.

20. From statement (1), the average could be 67, 68, or 69 depending on whether the four numbers are: (65, 66, x, 70), (65, 66, 70, 71), or (66, x, 70, 71). Statement (2) alone gives $x = 68$ which answers the question. The best choice is B.

21. From the figure, it follows that $x + y + (180 - z) + (180 - w) = 360$ which simplifies to $z = x + y - w$. Statement (1) is insufficient by itself, and (2) alone gives $z = x$ which does not give an explicit value for z. Statements (1) and (2) together give the answer, $z = 60$. The correct answer is C.

22. From the problem statement, $x^2 + y^2 = w^3 + z^2 + 1$, or $w^3 = x^2 + y^2 - z^2 - 1$. Using (1) in this gives $w^3 = 1$ from which $w = -1$; with (2) alone, $w^3 = 31 - z^2$, but this does not permit the unique determination of w. The best answer is A.

23. The problem can be rewritten into $x^2 = z^3 + (2x)(y + x - z)$. Using the first statement, the problem reduces to $x^2 = z^3$, but without the value of z, no value for x can be determined. Using statement (2) does not allow evaluation as no value for y or z is provided. Using both gives, $x^2 = 64$ from which $x = +8$ or -8 since no indication was given whether x is positive or negative. Choice E.

24. The expression to be evaluated can be rewritten as $(x+y)(x+y)/(x+y)(x-y)$ which simplifies to $(x+y)/(x-y)$. Statement (1) by itself is insufficient to answer the question. From (2), $7(x-y) = (x+y)$ from which $6x = 8y$ or $x = 4y/3$. Using this in the simplified expression gives: $[(4y/3) + y]/[(4y/3) - y] = (7y/3)/(y/3) = 7$. The best answer is B.

25. There is insufficient information in both statements as there is no way of determining areas of the unshaded regions other than BCD. The correct answer is E.

Section V: Problem Solving.

1. The combination of the two reductions means that the customer gets a total reduction of 35% on the retail price and thus pays 65% of the original price. This is 0.65(15.00) = $9.75, choice C.

2. The first $\frac{1}{4}$ mile costs $2.25, the next 4 miles (at $2 per mile) costs $8 and the final $\frac{1}{4}$ mile costs $0.50 for a total of $10.75, choice B.

3. Expansion of the expression gives $6 + 2 - 2\sqrt{12}$ which simplifies to $8 - 4\sqrt{3}$, that is, answer E.

4. The expression given can be factored into $(x + y)(x - y)/[2(x - y)^2]$ which simplifies to $(x + y)/[2(x - y)]$. From $x + y = 6(x - y)$, $(x + y)/(x - y) = 6$, and the expression reduces to $6/2 = 3$, choice D.

5. The problem is equivalent to 8.047 - 1.690 which gives 6.357, choice B.

6. The original cost of the stock was 50 x $75 or $3,750. After the stock split, Franklin had 100 shares and a 10% stock dividend increased his total holdings to 110 shares which sold at $80 a share = $8,800 for a net gain of $5,050; choice C.

7. Since the arcs AB, BC, and CD must be equal, each arc represents 60°. If lines are drawn from points B and C to the mid-point of AD at E, equilateral triangles, ABE, BCE, and CDE are created. If lines BF and BD are drawn, these three triangles are cut in half, forming six identical right triangles. Since ABCD consists of these six identical right triangles and the shaded area consists of three of these triangles, then the ratio of the areas must be $3/6 = \frac{1}{2}$, choice A.

8. The statement of the problem implies that a and c are prime numbers. If M is the number between a and c, then M is the average of a and c, and it follows that $a + c = 2M$. Since, for any three consecutive numbers, one of the three must be a multiple of 3 and at least one of the three must be a multiple of 2, then M must be both a multiple of 2 and 3 since both a and c are primes. M is thus a multiple of $2 \times 3 = 6$, and 2M, (i.e., a + c) is a multiple of 2×6 or 12, choice E.

9. It is clear from the figure, that the perimeter is made up of 4 quarter circles and 4 semi-circles, all with a radius equal to one-quarter of the distance between A and B or B and C. The perimeter is thus equivalent to the perimeter of 3 full circles of radius 2 which gives $3(2\pi R) = 12\pi$, choice E.

10. From the figure, it follows that $x + 2a + 2b = 180$. Since AB || CD, then we get the relationship, $3a = 180 - 3b$, from which $a + b = 60$. Using this in the first expression gives $x = 60$, choice B.

11. If five consecutive numbers have an average of 87, reducing each by 2 will reduce the average by the 2 as well to 85. Dividing each of these numbers by five will result in an average that is 1/5 as large, and 1/5 of 85 is 17, choice D.

12. For DC = 3, BC = 4, and AB = 12. Using the Pythagorean theorem with BC = 4 and DC = 3, BD works out to be 5. With this value and AB = 12, the Pythagorean theorem gives AD = 13, choice C.

13. The difference between the nth term and the next larger term is given by $(4[n + 1]^2 + 1) - (4n^2 + 1) = 4n^2 + 8n + 4 + 1 - 4n^2 - 1 = 8n + 4$, choice D.

14. If A represents the average daily sales figures during week 2, then, daily sales during week 3 must average 1.2A. As the difference from one week to the next is the same, 1.2A - A = 0.2A must represent the change for each week; the corresponding daily sales figures must be 0.8A in week 1 and 1.4A in week 4. The average for all four weeks is (0.8A + A + 1.2A + 1.4A)/4 = 1.1A. Since 1.1A must equal $3,300, then A = $3,000. The difference between week 1 and week 4 is 1.4A - 0.8A = 0.6A = (0.6)($3,000) = $1,800, choice B.

15. Using the expression, $12^* = \frac{1}{4}(10)(12)(14) = 420$. Similarly, $5^* = \frac{1}{4}(3)(5)(7) = 105/4$. $12^*/5^*$ becomes $420 \div 105/4 = 420(4)/105 = 16$, choice E.

16. Assuming that the first of the 17 numbers is A, then, the second is A + 1, the third, A + 2, ..., and the last, A + 16. The average of these numbers will be the 9th number, A + 8. For the new set of the numbers, the first number would be A + 20, the second, (A + 1) + 19, the third, (A + 2) + 18, ... , to (A + 16) + 4. Since each number in the new set is identical and equal to A + 20, it follows that the new set has an average of A + 20. The difference between the average of the new set, A + 20 and the former average, A + 8, is 12, choice C.

17. The comparison can be readily made by expressing each as the fourth root of a number, thus, $2^{\frac{3}{4}} = (2^3)^{\frac{1}{4}} = 8^{\frac{1}{4}}$; $3^{\frac{1}{2}} = (3^2)^{\frac{1}{4}} = 9^{\frac{1}{4}}$; and $4^{\frac{1}{4}}$. It follows that in increasing order, the values are $4^{\frac{1}{4}}$, $8^{\frac{1}{4}}$, $9^{\frac{1}{4}}$, corresponding to $4^{\frac{1}{4}}$, $2^{\frac{3}{4}}$, $3^{\frac{1}{2}}$, choice D.

18. From the first relationship, x must be 1, 2, 3, 4, or 5. From the second relationship, y^2 must be 4, 9, or 16, and y must be 2, 3, or 4. Of the choices offered, only D is not possible as the relationship can be rewritten, by dividing all terms by y, to become $2(x/y) < 2y - 9$. Since the right hand term is always negative for any allowable value of y, and left hand term is positive since x and y are both positive, the inequality is contradicted which is the choice required.

19. Grouping the fractions in groups of two, since 1/3 - 1/4 is positive, and 1/5 - 1/6 is positive, then S = a positive quantity plus a positive quantity plus 1/7 so S must be greater than 1/7. Grouping the same numbers as 1/3 + (-1/4 + 1/5) + (-1/6 + 1/7) gives S as equal to 1/3 plus two negative terms, and S must be less than 1/3. Choice C is the correct answer.

20. If N is rewritten as N = (999X + X) + (99Y + Y) + (9Z + Z) = 9(111X + 11Y + Z) + (X + Y + Z), it follows that X + Y + Z is the remainder after N is divided by 9. Since X, Y, and Z must be 1, 2, and 3 in some order, the remainder must be 1 + 2 + 3 = 6, which is choice C.

Section VI: Sentence Correction.

1. In the correct answer, C, the verb seems agrees with mayor, i.e., the nearer of its compound subjects correlated by neither ...nor. Choices A and D err in this agreement. Moreover, choices B, D, and E substitute or for nor.

2. The best answer, E, applies number to the count noun, phenomena. In choices A and B, amount (properly applicable to mass nouns like snow) incorrectly replaces number. Moreover, in choice A, the antecedent of the pronoun them is ambiguous, as is the antecedent of it in C and D.

3. The correct choice, A, clearly relates the introductory subordinate clause to the main clause. The use of inasmuch as in choice C is slightly stilted and indirect. Choice D is awkward and wordy. Choice E misrelates the subordinate clause beginning with because to the linking verb is. Choice B fails to clarify the logical relation between reacting and sodium.

4. The correct choice, D, relates the introductory infinitive phrase to librarian. In A, B, and C, this phrase is dangling. C and E split the second infinitive (to not keep). Moreover, in choices A, C, and E, desk should be plural to agree with readers.

5. In the correct choice, B, as, a conjunction, is followed by verb and subject in idiomatically inverted order. In A, as appears unidiomatically as a preposition. Choice E is awkward in word order, and done, in E, is redundant. Choices C and D misuse the preposition like as a conjunction.

6. The correct choice, A, contains the uninflected past participle of burst. In B, bust, is, of course, slang. In C, being that is a substandard idiom, as is being as in E.

7. The best choice, C, is preferable on grounds of diction to A, which contains the awkward dissimilar to. In B, D, and E, an adverbial clause incorrectly follows the linking verb (such is when definitions are not acceptable in formal contexts).

8. The correct answer, A, construes the collective noun faculty as singular (the faculty is acting as a unit). Choices B, C, and E are in error on this point. Moreover, liable in B, D, and E is substandard as a synonym for likely in this context.

9. In the correct choice, A, the indefinite pronoun neither agrees with the singular verb appears. D and E err in agreement. In C, the relative pronoun which incorrectly refers to the whole idea of the preceding clause. B must be faulted for its parenthetical placing of the phrase not surprisingly.

10. The correct answer, D, shows the acceptable level of diction. In A, exacerbated is a malapropism. In B and E, disinterested (as a synonym for uninterested) is a colloquialism, as is aggravated (for exasperated) in B and C.

11. The correct choice, B, idiomatically uses the past participle of prepare at the beginning of a participial phrase. In A, to be is redundant. In C and D, the present participle preparing makes no sense since the main verb is in the present tense. C and E introduce the colloquial usage of where for in which.

12. The correct choice, E, puts the subject (your) of the gerund sending in the possessive case. Moreover, masterfully in E is preferable to masterly as an adverb. B introduces a clause as the object of appreciate, but to do so is to introduce an inappropriate meaning of appreciate. Choice C is wordy.

13. In the correct choice, B, support agrees with the antecedent of who, which is representatives, not one. Moreover, in A, D, and E, the gerund ratifying is unidiomatically substituted for the noun.

14. The correct choice, E, is most concise. Choices B and D are wordy. Choice A omits the; choice C, the final of.

15. The correct answer, E, applies among to many anthropologists; between in B and C properly applies to only two. Moreover, in regards to in A and with regards to in C are nonstandard idioms. In D, with regard to is awkward.

16. In the correct answer, A, that introduces a noun clause ending in professions, a clause which acts as the subject of the sentence. Each of the other answer choices introduces a subordinate clause which has no grammatical relation to the rest of the sentence.

17. The correct answer, D, applies who to women (which, as a relative pronoun, is applied to things). B contains a redundant else; and both B and C omit a second have, since in B and C, either is placed before the verb. In E, either is placed in a position requiring a repetition of both who and the verb.

18. In the correct answer, B, the comparison, as successful as, is complete; and the subject of the elliptical clause is put in the subjective case: as successful as ... we (have been). Choice D introduces a new error in the illogical comparison between competitors, in the first part of the sentence, and our efforts.

19. The correct answer, B, co-ordinates the two main ideas of the statement in a compound-complex sentence. A and C cause the introductory participial phrase, isolated long enough, to dangle. A, D, and E close with a misrelated and vague participial phrase.

20. In the correct answer, C, the grammar reflects the plural number of emphases. B, D, and E assume that emphases is singular. Moreover, A and D introduce the wrong prepositional idiom of the verb derive.

21. The correct answer, C, introduces a noun clause following the linking verb is. Consequently, choice C avoids the substandard pattern, the ... reason ... is because ..., in A, B, and D. Moreover, this in A and E is ambiguous, as is its in D.

22. The correct choice, B, uses the perfect infinitive, to have had, called for by the sequence (the performance took place before the judging). B also avoids the illogical comparison of the absolute adjective perfect in A and D. Moreover, the preposition between indicates that the superlative forms in C and D are wrong, since only two gymnasts were competing.

23. In the correct choice, E, the less important idea in the statement is subordinated in a relative clause. This subordination is preferable to the awkward co-ordination of B, or to the subordination of the more important idea of the statement, in A. Moreover, even is best placed after spoken, as in E. In C, the parenthetical placement of the main clause is awkward. In D, the word order is quite confused.

24. The correct answer, E, exhibits parallel structure in its noun clause, which expresses futurity by means of would. A and B fail to introduce a noun clause to parallel that in the last clause of the sentence. C is wordy, and D is ambiguous and awkward.

25. The best choice, D, exhibits a double subjunctive. The first verb in the subjunctive mood, were, expresses a condition contrary to fact; second, the correlated verbs vindicate and sit are put in the subjunctive mood because of their position in a that clause following an expression of demand. On this basis, choices A, B, and C may be ruled out. In E, as in B, not only is misplaced. Moreover, the present perfect form have demanded in E is redundant.

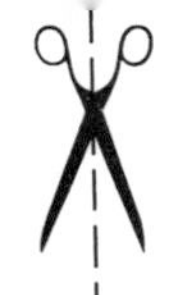

PASTEST

GMAT ANSWER SHEET: EXAM 1

NAME .... DATE ....

ADDRESS ....

....

SECTION 1	SECTION 2	SECTION 3	SECTION 4	SECTION 5	SECTION 6
1 A B C D E	1 A B C D E	1 A B C D E	1 A B C D E	1 A B C D E	1 A B C D E
2 A B C D E	2 A B C D E	2 A B C D E	2 A B C D E	2 A B C D E	2 A B C D E
3 A B C D E	3 A B C D E	3 A B C D E	3 A B C D E	3 A B C D E	3 A B C D E
4 A B C D E	4 A B C D E	4 A B C D E	4 A B C D E	4 A B C D E	4 A B C D E
5 A B C D E	5 A B C D E	5 A B C D E	5 A B C D E	5 A B C D E	5 A B C D E
6 A B C D E	6 A B C D E	6 A B C D E	6 A B C D E	6 A B C D E	6 A B C D E
7 A B C D E	7 A B C D E	7 A B C D E	7 A B C D E	7 A B C D E	7 A B C D E
8 A B C D E	8 A B C D E	8 A B C D E	8 A B C D E	8 A B C D E	8 A B C D E
9 A B C D E	9 A B C D E	9 A B C D E	9 A B C D E	9 A B C D E	9 A B C D E
10 A B C D E	10 A B C D E	10 A B C D E	10 A B C D E	10 A B C D E	10 A B C D E
11 A B C D E	11 A B C D E	11 A B C D E	11 A B C D E	11 A B C D E	11 A B C D E
12 A B C D E	12 A B C D E	12 A B C D E	12 A B C D E	12 A B C D E	12 A B C D E
13 A B C D E	13 A B C D E	13 A B C D E	13 A B C D E	13 A B C D E	13 A B C D E
14 A B C D E	14 A B C D E	14 A B C D E	14 A B C D E	14 A B C D E	14 A B C D E
15 A B C D E	15 A B C D E	15 A B C D E	15 A B C D E	15 A B C D E	15 A B C D E
16 A B C D E	16 A B C D E	16 A B C D E	16 A B C D E	16 A B C D E	16 A B C D E
17 A B C D E	17 A B C D E	17 A B C D E	17 A B C D E	17 A B C D E	17 A B C D E
18 A B C D E	18 A B C D E	18 A B C D E	18 A B C D E	18 A B C D E	18 A B C D E
19 A B C D E	19 A B C D E	19 A B C D E	19 A B C D E	19 A B C D E	19 A B C D E
20 A B C D E	20 A B C D E	20 A B C D E	20 A B C D E	20 A B C D E	20 A B C D E
21 A B C D E	21 A B C D E	21 A B C D E	21 A B C D E	21 A B C D E	21 A B C D E
22 A B C D E	22 A B C D E	22 A B C D E	22 A B C D E	22 A B C D E	22 A B C D E
23 A B C D E	23 A B C D E	23 A B C D E	23 A B C D E	23 A B C D E	23 A B C D E
24 A B C D E	24 A B C D E	24 A B C D E	24 A B C D E	24 A B C D E	24 A B C D E
25 A B C D E	25 A B C D E	25 A B C D E	25 A B C D E	25 A B C D E	25 A B C D E
26 A B C D E	26 A B C D E	26 A B C D E	26 A B C D E	26 A B C D E	26 A B C D E
27 A B C D E	27 A B C D E	27 A B C D E	27 A B C D E	27 A B C D E	27 A B C D E
28 A B C D E	28 A B C D E	28 A B C D E	28 A B C D E	28 A B C D E	28 A B C D E
29 A B C D E	29 A B C D E	29 A B C D E	29 A B C D E	29 A B C D E	29 A B C D E
30 A B C D E	30 A B C D E	30 A B C D E	30 A B C D E	30 A B C D E	30 A B C D E
31 A B C D E	31 A B C D E	31 A B C D E	31 A B C D E	31 A B C D E	31 A B C D E
32 A B C D E	32 A B C D E	32 A B C D E	32 A B C D E	32 A B C D E	32 A B C D E
33 A B C D E	33 A B C D E	33 A B C D E	33 A B C D E	33 A B C D E	33 A B C D E
34 A B C D E	34 A B C D E	34 A B C D E	34 A B C D E	34 A B C D E	34 A B C D E
35 A B C D E	35 A B C D E	35 A B C D E	35 A B C D E	35 A B C D E	35 A B C D E

PASTEST

GMAT ANSWER SHEET: EXAM 2

SURNAME	INITIALS	DATE

SECTION 1	SECTION 2	SECTION 3	SECTION 4	SECTION 5	SECTION 6
1 A B C D E	1 A B C D E	1 A B C D E	1 A B C D E	1 A B C D E	1 A B C D E
2 A B C D E	2 A B C D E	2 A B C D E	2 A B C D E	2 A B C D E	2 A B C D E
3 A B C D E	3 A B C D E	3 A B C D E	3 A B C D E	3 A B C D E	3 A B C D E
4 A B C D E	4 A B C D E	4 A B C D E	4 A B C D E	4 A B C D E	4 A B C D E
5 A B C D E	5 A B C D E	5 A B C D E	5 A B C D E	5 A B C D E	5 A B C D E
6 A B C D E	6 A B C D E	6 A B C D E	6 A B C D E	6 A B C D E	6 A B C D E
7 A B C D E	7 A B C D E	7 A B C D E	7 A B C D E	7 A B C D E	7 A B C D E
8 A B C D E	8 A B C D E	8 A B C D E	8 A B C D E	8 A B C D E	8 A B C D E
9 A B C D E	9 A B C D E	9 A B C D E	9 A B C D E	9 A B C D E	9 A B C D E
10 A B C D E	10 A B C D E	10 A B C D E	10 A B C D E	10 A B C D E	10 A B C D E
11 A B C D E	11 A B C D E	11 A B C D E	11 A B C D E	11 A B C D E	11 A B C D E
12 A B C D E	12 A B C D E	12 A B C D E	12 A B C D E	12 A B C D E	12 A B C D E
13 A B C D E	13 A B C D E	13 A B C D E	13 A B C D E	13 A B C D E	13 A B C D E
14 A B C D E	14 A B C D E	14 A B C D E	14 A B C D E	14 A B C D E	14 A B C D E
15 A B C D E	15 A B C D E	15 A B C D E	15 A B C D E	15 A B C D E	15 A B C D E
16 A B C D E	16 A B C D E	16 A B C D E	16 A B C D E	16 A B C D E	16 A B C D E
17 A B C D E	17 A B C D E	17 A B C D E	17 A B C D E	17 A B C D E	17 A B C D E
18 A B C D E	18 A B C D E	18 A B C D E	18 A B C D E	18 A B C D E	18 A B C D E
19 A B C D E	19 A B C D E	19 A B C D E	19 A B C D E	19 A B C D E	19 A B C D E
20 A B C D E	20 A B C D E	20 A B C D E	20 A B C D E	20 A B C D E	20 A B C D E
21 A B C D E	21 A B C D E	21 A B C D E	21 A B C D E	21 A B C D E	21 A B C D E
22 A B C D E	22 A B C D E	22 A B C D E	22 A B C D E	22 A B C D E	22 A B C D E
23 A B C D E	23 A B C D E	23 A B C D E	23 A B C D E	23 A B C D E	23 A B C D E
24 A B C D E	24 A B C D E	24 A B C D E	24 A B C D E	24 A B C D E	24 A B C D E
25 A B C D E	25 A B C D E	25 A B C D E	25 A B C D E	25 A B C D E	25 A B C D E
26 A B C D E	26 A B C D E	26 A B C D E	26 A B C D E	26 A B C D E	26 A B C D E
27 A B C D E	27 A B C D E	27 A B C D E	27 A B C D E	27 A B C D E	27 A B C D E
28 A B C D E	28 A B C D E	28 A B C D E	28 A B C D E	28 A B C D E	28 A B C D E
29 A B C D E	29 A B C D E	29 A B C D E	29 A B C D E	29 A B C D E	29 A B C D E
30 A B C D E	30 A B C D E	30 A B C D E	30 A B C D E	30 A B C D E	30 A B C D E
31 A B C D E	31 A B C D E	31 A B C D E	31 A B C D E	31 A B C D E	31 A B C D E
32 A B C D E	32 A B C D E	32 A B C D E	32 A B C D E	32 A B C D E	32 A B C D E
33 A B C D E	33 A B C D E	33 A B C D E	33 A B C D E	33 A B C D E	33 A B C D E
34 A B C D E	34 A B C D E	34 A B C D E	34 A B C D E	34 A B C D E	34 A B C D E
35 A B C D E	35 A B C D E	35 A B C D E	35 A B C D E	35 A B C D E	35 A B C D E